D0813570

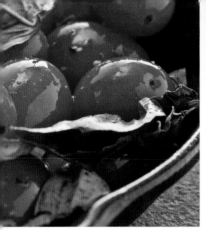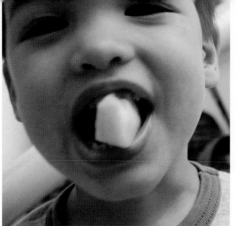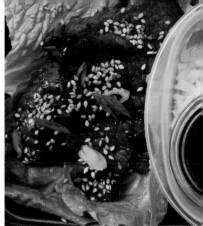

what chefs feed their kids

RECIPES AND TECHNIQUES FOR CULTIVATING A LOVE OF GOOD FOOD

FANAE AARON

FOOD PHOTOGRAPHY BY VIKTOR BUDNIK

LYONS PRESS
GUILFORD, CONNECTICUT
An imprint of Globe Pequot Press

for cody

To buy books in quantity for corporate use
or incentives, call **(800) 962–0973**
or e-mail **premiums@GlobePequot.com.**

Lyons Press is an imprint of Globe Pequot Press.

Food photography by Viktor Budnik
Text design: Nancy Freeborn
Layout artists: Sue Murray and Melissa Evarts
Project editor: Gregory Hyman

Library of Congress Cataloging-in-Publication Data is available on file.

ISBN 978-0-7627-6095-4

Printed in the U.S.A.

10 9 8 7 6 5 4 3 2

acknowledgments

I want to acknowledge and thank my husband, Flint, for his patience, his kindness, and his love, and my son Cody, who has been a wonder in both our lives—he is also mostly a pleasure to feed. In writing this book I have come to know so many people. I want to thank the community of people who have been so helpful—all the chefs who have participated in the project for sharing not only their personal recipes but their personal stories with me. I know this topic is as important to all of them as it is to me. I want to thank my dedicated foodie friend Kelley King and my friend Piper Bridges-Fila. I also want to thank Leslie Nichols for all of her insight and encouragement. I want to also thank my friend Mary Ann Marino, who jumped in to help on this book when it was only an idea. I can't thank Sue Bell and all the kids at her school, Giggles and Grass Stains, enough for enthusiastically tasting food prepared from the recipes in this book that I would make and bring in for snacks. I want to acknowledge and thank my agent Jenni Ferrari-Adler and the team at Globe Pequot Press, including my editors Mary Norris and Lara Asher, who have been so encouraging, helpful, and supportive.

contents

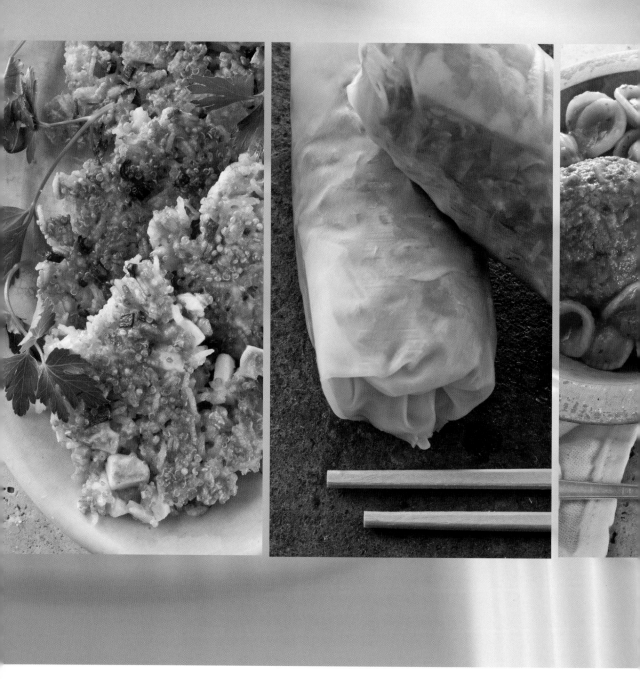

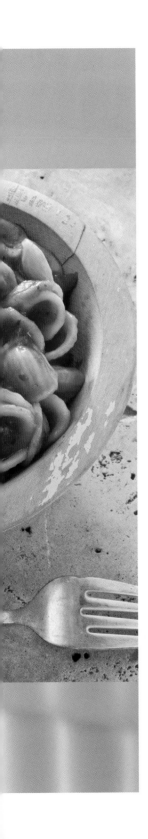

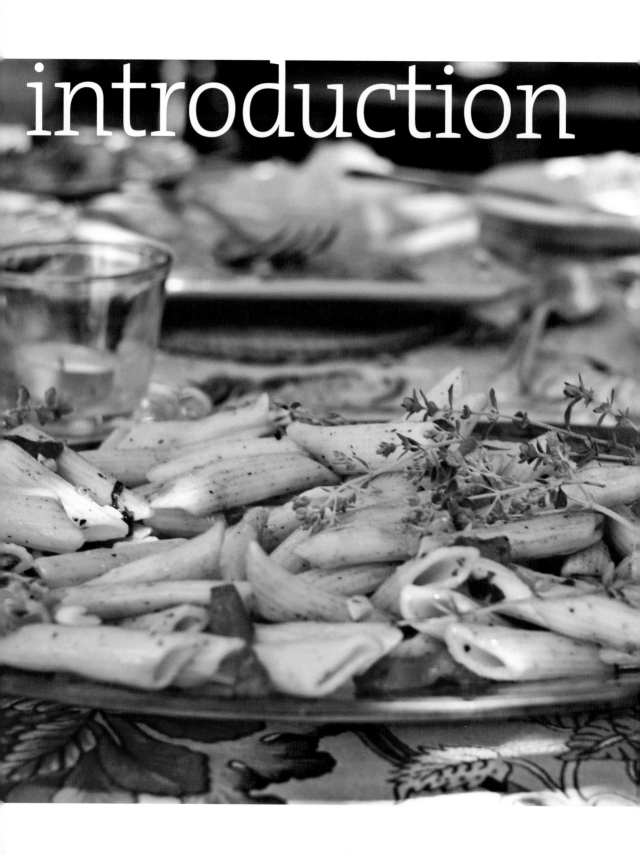

introduction

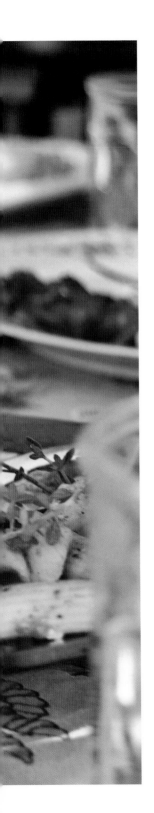

When it came time to start feeding my son, Cody, solid foods, like most parents I trooped to the store and stocked up on jars of baby food in a variety of flavors. But then when the time came, I popped open a jar and it just didn't seem that appetizing. Instead, I simply gave Cody some sweet potato that I was eating, then some mashed ripe avocado. I liked that he and I could eat the same thing. Even at the very beginning, we could sit and enjoy a meal together. I knew that what he was eating was good, because I was tasting it myself. But I didn't know where to go from there. I had only rudimentary cooking skills and didn't know what to do to add variety, or even if I should. It was easy to mash some sweet potato with a fork, but I didn't know if I should mix it up and try new things or stick to what Cody liked. I wondered if there was a way to feed kids that both nourishes and stimulates them. Our brains are wired to burst to life with new sensations. They light up and chemicals are released in our brains as we experience the pleasure and delight of something new and interesting. Cody did seem to get very excited about the physical sensation of food in his mouth and a spoon in his hand, and he was very pleased when the two met.

I wondered: Would a child raised by chefs enjoy eating even vegetables, which most kids detest and refuse? What kinds of things do chefs do to introduce their children to eating, and are they able to stimulate curiosity about new foods? Do their kids pick out the smallest speck of parsley and call foods "icky" and "gross," just like other children do?

For chefs, every meal is a new beginning—an adventure—and that attitude translates to how they feed their kids. I interviewed lots of chefs all around the country for this book and collected their voices and ideas together. This book illustrates their strategies and their attitudes; it's not just about cooking for your kids. I now enjoy cooking family meals, but the techniques are the same for eating out.

It's about how we can educate kids and eventually enable them, when they are old enough, to make better choices for nourishing themselves.

The recipes in this book are meant to be served as meals for the whole family. Here, the purees are a pared-down part of an overall recipe that the whole family can eat, with suggestions for additions or modifications for older children and adults. Also, the foods in the beginning are more rudimentary and simpler to prepare than the recipes later in the book. Lots of the recipes can be tackled together, with young children doing the measuring and pouring and, later in the book, older children learning about transforming ingredients and the magic of assembling them to make a complete dish together.

The book is organized in chapters by age, recognizing that there are ways that babies and younger children prefer to eat that are different from the kinds of foods that older children gravitate toward. I've tested all these recipes myself and tried to explain some of the trickier parts of recipes and why they are tricky. Some of the ingredients I'd never heard of before—*tamarind? Is it a paste or a fruit?*—and it was a bit of an adventure finding them.

"When people enter the kitchen, they often drag their childhood in with them," says novelist and food writer Laurie Colwin in her book *Home Cooking*. I remember reading her books of essays when Cody was an infant, during his naps. When I look back at those days, I realize that those sweet potatoes became the basis for our relationship and how we experience a meal—cooking together, sharing food together, eating together. We had fun, we learned a lot, and sometimes we struggled. This early foundation still underlies the way we eat and share a meal. Food writer M. F. K. Fisher summed it up when she said, "It seems to me that our three basic needs, for food and security and love, are so mixed and mingled and entwined that we cannot straightly think of one without the others."

recipe list

adolescence { ages eight to eleven }

infancy

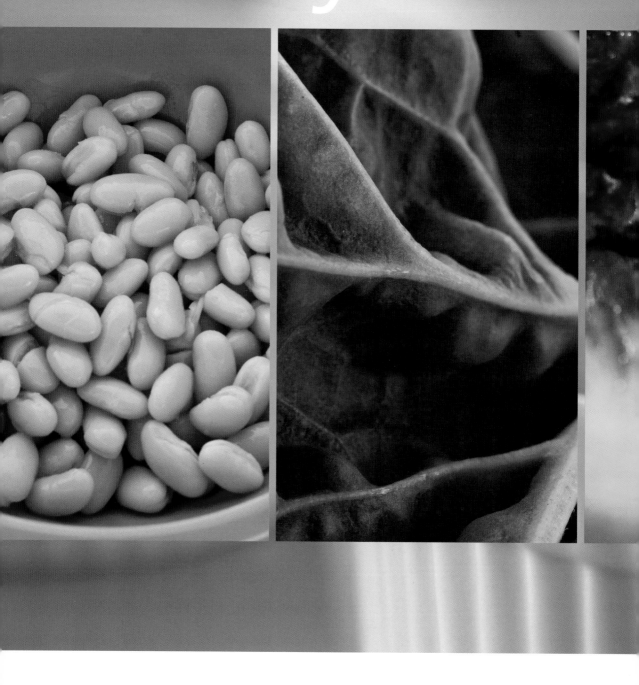

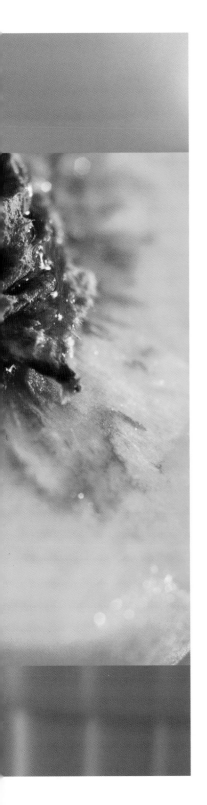

A FOUNDATION OF SIMPLE FOOD

ages zero to one

Food is one of the keys to the world of pleasure and adventure in life, according to the chefs I interviewed for this book. It stimulates the senses unlike anything else—and we can impart a desire for that stimulation, as well as a curiosity about new experiences, early in our children's lives by serving them a broad range of colorful, flavorful foods that they can experience with all their senses. Food is about so much more than taste, especially for infants. It's a whole new world for an infant to start eating solid foods, foods that the grown-ups have been eating. Rich with sensory stimulation, food excites infants with its vibrant colors and savory smells. They enjoy putting it in their mouths, rolling it around and tasting it, or just squishing it in their hands and mushing it around the table.

When Do Babies First Experience Flavor?

A baby first experiences flavor in the womb, where taste buds initially develop. "Nourishment and taste buds start in the womb, so what a mother eats is what's in the placenta," says Sally Kravich, a natural health expert. Remarkably, a fetus at fifteen weeks has taste buds that resemble an adult's, and before the end of the first trimester, a baby tastes the flavors of foods by sucking, swallowing, and even smelling amniotic fluid. After birth, a breast-fed baby receives a variety of flavors through the taste and aroma of breast milk, which is constantly changing. Because the foods we eat flavor our breast milk, a breast-fed baby becomes accustomed to those flavors and their variety. "I've never censored or changed my eating, especially while breast-feeding," says Chef Ana Sortun, who wanted her daughter, Siena, to grow to enjoy the same foods she eats. Sortun, who is the chef/owner of the award-winning Oleana Restaurant in Boston, ignored the recommendations of some pediatricians to restrict her diet and avoid a whole host of foods, including garlic, cabbage, and broccoli, while breast-feeding her newborn. "I think from even before she was eating herself, she had a sense of flavor and spices."

The flavor of formula, on the other hand, is bland, sweet, and unvarying from bottle to bottle. It leads to early conditioning for bland, one-note foods. While breast-feeding is far better for infants for many reasons, not every chef's child included in this book was nursed, and feeding infants formula does not at all mean that ultimately they won't eat well as they get older. Nursing a child, as beneficial overall as it is, is just one of many opportunities to teach a child to eat well and acclimate her palate.

Building Blocks of Flavor

When it came time to introduce solids to their infants, the chefs profiled here all started out feeding their kids a foundation of fresh vegetables and simple foods, like building blocks of flavor. Frank Proto, executive chef at Marc Murphy's Benchmarc group of restaurants in and around New York, takes a simple approach, pureeing steamed vegetables. He says, "I want them to experience the pure flavor of foods as they are." Colby Garrelts, chef and owner with his wife, Megan, of Bluestem restaurant in Kansas City, makes purees from fresh vegetables as well, and also offers pureed chicken soup. Chef B. T. Nguyen of Restaurant BT in Tampa points out that babies have palates that are pure and uncontaminated. They need to be given those clean and fresh foods first, she says. Other chefs mention roasting vegetables or fruits to concentrate and sweeten their flavors, and gradually adding another layer of flavor, like lemon or basil.

Perhaps the easiest time to feed a child is at the beginning, when he first starts to eat solid food. My son, Cody, was open and adventurous in the beginning because he had been watching me and my husband, Flint, eat and wanted to participate. The food went into his mouth and, for the most part, didn't come back out. He rolled the food around in his mouth but didn't intentionally reject it—that didn't occur until later.

Taking cues from the chefs I spoke with, when I began to feed Cody solid food, I stayed away from the rice cereal so many books recommended. I didn't want to celebrate such an event with the blandest and least exciting food ever created. It's best to start slow with solid foods and make them liquid and smooth, so I chose to start with a pureed banana. Then I moved on to pureed apple and sweet potato—foods I love, with color and texture. I added other vegetables, like green beans, peas, squash, and carrots. I also made purees from fruits such as peaches, plums, avocados, and apricots. And I mixed breast milk into the purees both to thin them and to help Cody adjust to the new flavors. For babies who are being fed formula, mixing that familiar formula in with new purees will help them acclimate to those new flavors.

I spaced out those first foods to watch for allergic reactions. Cynthia Epps, an infant-feeding specialist in Los Angeles, where we live, recommends doing this, especially if there is a family history of allergies. I began combining foods to keep things interesting. I mixed up Cody's food a lot, and while we had some staples we repeated regularly and frequently, there was always something new on the menu. I often had him on my hip while we were in the kitchen mixing and mashing, giving him tastes of food as I tasted it while cooking. I tried to follow Cody's cues and be sensitive to reflux, gas, and elimination issues, which are common when babies first begin eating solids. I avoided raw fish, like sushi, which can have harmful bacteria, and spicy foods.

I quickly began experimenting. I mixed baked apple puree with herbs like rosemary, tarragon, or

COLBY AND MEGAN GARRELTS have their own restaurant in Kansas City, Missouri, called Bluestem. Colby is the executive chef, and Megan is the pastry chef. Colby was listed as one of the Best New Chefs in 2005 by *Food & Wine*. He was nominated by the James Beard Foundation for Best Chef Midwest Region for 2007 and 2008. For the restaurant, they source their organic produce and meats locally. They serve progressive American farm-to-table fine dining, and they opened a casual lounge next door that serves beautiful bistro french fries with truffle oil, parsley, and cheese. Their daughter, Madi, spends lots of time at the restaurant and knows just where the chocolate bin is in the area where Megan bakes. "I go back there and her cheeks are full of chocolate," says Colby. "She'll go to the kitchen and the cooks will give her things all the time. She's tasting things all the time. She will definitely know food."

Megan Garrelts and daughter Madi : BONJWING LEE

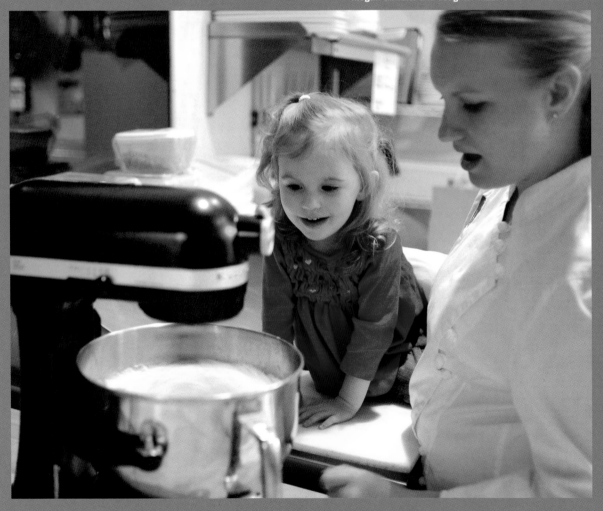

thyme, playing up savory flavors instead of sweet. I mashed carrots and butternut squash together and alternated days of kale and spinach, which I made the way I like them, with olive oil and garlic, so we could eat together. I wanted Cody to eat dark leafy greens, which I love. Cody was born in late March, so when I started giving him solid foods, it was late summer and early autumn. Stone fruits like peaches and plums were fresh at the market, and I roasted them and mixed them into cereals and oatmeal that we all enjoyed together.

After Cody adjusted to eating purees, I began to vary them by texture, color, and flavor and learned from Diane Forley, chef and co-owner with her chef husband, Michael Otsuka, of Flourish Bakery in Scarsdale, New York, to make them flavorful instead of tasteless and boring. She makes fresh soup stock—squash, turnip, rutabaga, and chicken—and adds fresh herbs. "Adding herbs is how I make my food flavorful," she says. "I also use onion to add flavor. Why do people think kids should eat food that's bland? Prepared baby foods are bland. I don't know why there's an assumption that kids don't have taste buds."

Proto agrees. "My daughter loves miso soup," he says. "She loves it! Who would think that a kid would like miso soup?"

Marcia Pelchat, a biopsychologist at the Monell Chemical Senses Center in Philadelphia, explains that infants prefer a salt solution to plain water as early as five months and will enjoy soups and broths.

Most chefs make and keep stocks at home to incorporate in everyday cooking as both a way to make food flavorful and to get multiple meals from one dish. Premium ingredients can be expensive, and getting the most from them is a good way to economize. Linton Hopkins, executive chef at Restaurant Eugene in Atlanta, makes quick stocks from leftover chicken and bones while he's cleaning up dishes. He'll use that stock for a rice and chicken dish the following night. He'll make a quick broth out of the unused vegetable parts like leek tops. "To me, making a stock is like making a tea," Hopkins says. "People get scared of stocks, but those are the juices that make our cooking better, I think."

Introducing Your Baby to Spoon Feeding

Epps considers infants' oral and tactile development as well as guidelines established by the American Dietetic Association when offering advice on how to go about helping infants learn to eat from a spoon.

The first thing I do is to slowly bring a spoonful of puree toward the child. Children will reach out for it on their own because, developmentally, they are exploring the world through their hands at this age. They'll take the spoon if it's pointing in the right direction and if it's put close to their hands, and they will put it by themselves right into their mouth.

This gets children to participate from the very beginning. When they are feeding themselves, they will naturally eat slower than an adult would feed them and they will intuitively eat an amount that is right for them. Adults who feed infants will be inclined to feed them a whole jar or whole bowlful of food, and that's probably too much for them. At first, the purees should be very liquid and roll easily off the spoon—at eight to ten months you can start to make them thicker. A child at six to twelve months is going through a stage of oral and tactile development that involves passing toys from hand to hand. Giving them the spoon makes their meals part of that development, and it's fun for them.

When babies take the spoon themselves, they will naturally chew on it with their gums and use more chewing pressure than if they were being fed. Allow them to take a spoon and chew and crush on it while they are eating. If, for a few seconds, they get to suck and chew and crush on the spoon, they slow down their eating and become patient. This does two things simultaneously. First, it teaches the child to eat slowly instead of grab food and gulp it down, and second, it lowers the risk of choking because the baby's mouth is developing a chew, crush, swallow, chew, crush, swallow pattern of eating. When an adult feeds a baby, they likely don't leave the spoon in her mouth to give her the opportunity to chew on it, so the baby just swallows the food.

If you allow babies that step of using their mouth to crush on the spoon with their gums, by the time they start to fully feed themselves at ten to twelve months, because they have learned that chewing is part of eating, the risk of choking later when they are eating pieces of food instead of puree is lowered.

The First Bite

Feeding children requires creativity, patience, persistence, and caring, and most children need to be given more than one opportunity to embrace a new food. While Cody was never terribly difficult about trying new foods, I was told many times not to assume he didn't like something until I'd fed it to him a few times. Some babies are slower to take to solid foods; they may have trouble learning to swallow or might be picky from the get-go. Don't give up. Move at a pace that is comfortable for your child and keep trying different foods to find ones he likes. I found myself surprised by many of the foods Cody ended up enjoying.

The first solid food Colby Garrelts gave Madi, his daughter, was carrots. "They are naturally sweeter. We figured she would go towards that first." He was surprised that the vegetables seemed to be the things she liked best. She likes squashes, spinach, carrots, and broccoli. She loves broccoli. "Broccoli stems are sweet," adds chef and cookbook author Peter Berley, and he peels the tough outer skin off and cooks the stems along with the florets.

It is especially important to give picky infants positive experiences with food. I sometimes had to play detective with Cody to figure out which foods he was adverse to and why, and which ones he naturally liked. I built flavor bases from there, giving him a variety that I think helped expand his diet later on. Also, at this early age a different preparation can make a food appetizing. Some foods, such as cabbage and asparagus, have sulfides in them and when cooked can smell bad to children who are sensitive to odors.

Chef, restaurateur, and food scientist Jimmy Schmidt discovered this with his son, Mike, who has difficulties with the aromas of certain foods. "If you look at asparagus, it's a great example because with raw asparagus, the sulfides are not as exposed and aromatic. When you cook it, it tends to get a little stinky. We're used to it, because as adults we like asparagus cooked and we are used to seeing it around. Just from a sheer aroma sense, you smell a raw asparagus and you smell a cooked asparagus, they smell quite different," he explains. "Mike's more open to raw than he is to cooked in the vegetable family. Even when he was a baby, he didn't like pureed peas and stuff like that."

Infants, who have a strong sense of smell, will judge a food on the spoon from a foot away and determine whether or not it's appealing to them. Asparagus, cabbage, broccoli, and cauliflower can be smelly when cooked and served warm. It is possible to cook them so they are soft but serve them cold to minimize their aromas. But even some hearty eaters will ease into eating slowly. As an infant, Cody would never just dig in to a plate of food unless it was a dish he'd had before and recognized. Given a few minutes, he'd take a bite and eventually finish what was on his plate.

I always made sure to give Cody a taste of what we were eating when we ate together. It has established a close bond between us that continues to evolve to this day. Sometimes he takes a bite of a particular food and doesn't like it, but he trusts me enough to take a taste because I have always been sensitive to his eating needs.

"The very first bite for Sasha is a difficult one. She never reacts 100 percent immediately. However, after a bite or two, then, it's like you open up the mouth. At first, she has a squeamish face, then slowly she feels like the comfort zone has arrived. You distract her. Distraction is very important. She needs to be focused. Babies are so busy with everything—if you don't make her focus, baby will not eat."

—Piero Selvaggio, owner of Valentino restaurants in Los Angeles and Las Vegas

Exposing a baby to a wide variety of foods, and consistently adding new foods, helps her eat broadly later as a preschooler and even as an adult. "Children of picky parents, parents who eat a narrow diet, end up just not being familiar with a lot of foods, and all things being equal, familiar foods are liked better than novel foods," says Pelchat. Chef Diane Forley confirms this when she says, "I think we set up and establish cravings in kids by serving certain types of food all the time. We get used to them."

Eat Healthy from the Start

It's easier to give your child a balanced and varied diet later on if you are eating that way while you are pregnant and breast-feeding. The early experience of the flavor of vegetables and other healthy foods has been found to familiarize babies with them, increasing the likelihood that they will accept those foods later when they begin eating them as solids. I saw it as an opportunity to begin building a foundation for Cody to enjoy a healthy, varied diet including vegetables.

Epps teaches her clients to begin feeding infants their first solids with a rotation of green and yellow vegetables and suggests serving fruits only occasionally. Even though so many pediatricians advocate starting with rice cereal mixed with fruit, she points out that rice cereal with fruit is a high-glycemic food. High-glycemic foods cause the blood sugar to rise quickly. Most fast foods are high-glycemic foods because of the added sugars they contain, and anything with the ingredient high-fructose corn syrup is high glycemic. By comparison, proteins, fats, grains, and nonstarchy or sweet vegetables don't impact blood sugar. Getting infants acclimated to eating high-glycemic foods sets them off on the wrong path, toward craving sweet foods. She suggests emphasizing vegetables and then rotating in different whole grains.

Epps proposes starting first with peas, then adding yams and summer squashes like zucchini, then adding a serving of apple before going back to peas again. She also advises staying away from sweetening vegetables or grains with fruits and instead letting those foods have their pure flavor. She recommends small portions, no bigger than the size of the baby's fist. Progressing this way prepares the infant's palate for accepting vegetables and makes it easier later to serve them as finger foods to a toddler, who becomes more difficult to feed.

The biggest problem with feeding children later on as toddlers and preschoolers is getting them to eat foods they are not familiar with—this can be anything that's new, like an avocado or ethnic dishes with unique flavors. Pelchat talks about the benefit of exposing kids to new foods and flavors, both to build familiarity with lots of foods and textures and also to build a tolerance for trying new foods. Scientific

PIERO SELVAGGIO has three grown sons—Giorgio, Giampiero, and Tancredi—and a new young daughter, Sasha. He is the owner of the fine Italian restaurants Valentino and Posto in Los Angeles and Valentino Las Vegas, at the Venetian Hotel in Las Vegas. His restaurant Valentino received the James Beard Award for Outstanding Service in 1996, and the award for wine in 1994. *Wine Spectator* magazine named Valentino one of the top four restaurants in the country in 1996 and again in 2000, and has given its Grand Award for wine to the restaurant every year since 1981. In 1997, the Italian magazine *Gambero Rosso* named Valentino the finest Italian restaurant in the world. Selvaggio was born in Modica, Sicily, and makes his home with his new family in Los Angeles. "I have something I could never have imagined could change my life so sweetly," says Selvaggio of having another child after his three sons were grown. "I couldn't imagine the journey. Interestingly enough, it has been a journey that has taught me a lot. For example, this morning, the highlight of my morning: I took her to the park and put her in the swing because she is a big girl, but the highlight was I made her a one-egg omelette with kale."

literature supports the idea that there is a window of opportunity to introduce children to novel foods that probably closes after they are weaned and before they turn two. Once that window closes, it becomes much harder to condition children to want to eat new things.

"It's important to begin a child with a healthy diet; you start a child not the wrong way but the right way. You put more care into building their taste buds for healthy foods and learning the balance of eating greens and of eating fruit and of eating healthy overall. The earlier you start training your child that this is the way to do things, the better it is," says Piero Selvaggio, chef and owner of Valentino restaurants in Los Angeles and Las Vegas.

"I never really put effort or so much thinking into eating healthy because where I was brought up, in my country, Vietnam, everything is organic and fresh and we don't have processed foods or canned foods. It is still in my mind and on my palate," says Nguyen. "So, I never bought baby food; I made baby food for my daughter. And the meals I made were always balanced. I would make dishes from a protein, a vegetable, and a starch. I would make her a dish of rice, chicken, and carrots, or I would make a variety of beef, rice, potato, and vegetable. I would cook it and then blend it, and if it needed, I put a little bit of milk in just for the consistency."

Part of eating healthy is eating broadly. "There's a lot of variety of foods around, all the time," says Sortun. Colby Garrelts says Madi, his daughter, spends a ton of time at their restaurant, where there are always lots of different things being cooked. "Madi

has known all the cooks and our general manager since she was born. She'll go to the back of the restaurant in the kitchen and the boys will give her things all the time; she's tasting things all the time and I hope she has a great palate. I thought about this a ton when she was first born. Kids here don't because most Americans don't eat this way, but in Vietnam for example infants grow up with fish sauce and curries."

Exposing children broadly includes keeping them around while you are cooking and also while you are eating, surrounding them with the aromas of what you are eating. "Siena, my daughter, is always in the kitchen with me when I am doing stuff," says Sortun. "Madi smells the food, that's a big deal too," adds Colby Garrelts.

try to avoid too many sweet flavors

Babies are naturally inclined to prefer sweet flavors and tend to initially reject sour and bitter flavors, so they may have a tougher time with savory vegetables. Children generally favor those fruits and vegetables that contain the most carbohydrates and sugars, such as potatoes, peas, bananas, and apples. It is believed that the preference for sweet flavors is biologically a protective function—plants with bitter and sour flavors are more likely to be poisonous or contain toxins. Repeated exposure helps kids get accustomed to those flavors and makes it easier for them to enjoy those nutritious vegetables that fall into this flavor range when they are older. Kravich says human beings naturally have a sweet tooth, and sweet is the strongest taste: "If children have been given sweets and haven't been properly introduced to foods in the weaning process in infancy or predominantly given sweet foods as infants, they're going to develop more of that sweet tooth."

on eating meat

Infants can begin to eat meat as early as eight to nine months of age. Megan Garrelts wanted her daughter, Madi, to eat meat because it contains protein and iron that she thought were important for nutrition. "In the beginning, we couldn't get her to eat meat at all," Megan says. "She would eat other things for protein, but it wasn't the same in our eyes. Then, we were having a bone-in rib eye for dinner, and she just picked the bone up off Colby's plate and started chewing on it because our dog had a bone and she was imitating the dog. From that day, instantly, all she wanted was steak. She was sucking on the meat and the bone and we thought 'oh my god, this is good.'"

Meat can be pureed like other foods, and it's easiest if it's mixed with a soup or a vegetable with a high water content, like tomato. "Most kids seem to like chicken more than anything because it's got a more mild flavor," says Colby Garrelts. Cody loved lamb and other roasted meats, and early on we were eating robustly flavored stews. I loved cooking those foods with him because we could casually prepare everything early in the day and have dinner ready without much immediate predinner preparation. It's also great to come home hungry to a house filled with the aromas of cooking.

the skinny on fat

Healthy babies are born fat. Fat comprises up to 14 percent of their body weight, half of which accumulates in the last five weeks in the womb. Baby fat is evenly distributed just under the skin, unlike adult fat, which accumulates internally around the organs. Healthy babies need fat to keep them warm and, even more important, for brain development and growth, which occur at a remarkable rate all through the first year of life. Seventy-four percent of a baby's energy in the first year of life is devoted to brain development, and that energy comes from fat. Skinny babies often do not flourish because the fatty acids meant for brain development are being used to keep them warm instead. Many of the developmental delays premature babies experience are due to lack of fat.

Healthy infants will continue to accumulate fat up to four times their birth amount during the first year of life. During this year most pediatricians advise giving infants full-fat dairy products, switching to low fat only after the first birthday.

But as children grow and develop, excess body fat causes problems. Sadly, children younger than six have been found to have fatty streaks on their arteries and some narrowing of the coronary arteries. Overweight infants are more likely to become overweight toddlers and stay overweight into adulthood. Studies show that the tipping point that determines obesity can occur as early as when infants are first learning what and how much to eat. Staying away from processed foods and eating healthy foods are critical for infants to learn to eat properly.

Allergies

Food allergies in infants can appear as cold symptoms such as a runny nose, itchy eyes, and a cough, or a rash. Highly allergenic foods include peanuts, milk, and eggs. Epps notes that it's important to remember that an infant's digestive system is different from an adult's. Infants are growing so quickly that the breast milk they consume goes straight into their bloodstream and is immediately used for tissue growth. The digestive system is very sensitive in the first twelve to fourteen months while it is maturing. Epps stresses that highly allergenic food like dairy, including yogurt, shouldn't be given to infants before their system matures, because early exposure to dairy products may actually create an allergic reaction.

Kravich says that children who seem to be chronically congested or who get sick with lots of runny noses, coughs, and colds may not be digesting wheat and dairy foods well. She says eating a fruit or vegetable with foods like starches, dairy, and proteins helps digestion. It's easy to give crackers, Cheerios, and pasta to children, but those foods alone, especially if not whole grain versions, are what Kravich calls "gluey" and "sticky" in the digestive system. She says, "It's like a glue, and it gets built up and it doesn't move through the digestive tract."

"Italians eat tomato with mozzarella; the Portuguese might have pear with a sheep's milk cheese. I started looking at how people eat things, and I realized that when I combine these live foods with dairy, I can digest it better and it doesn't produce mucous," says Kravich. She adds that cheese

"Food is family. There's a culture with Southern food that is all about family, very similar to the European cultures like the Italian culture and the Jewish close-knit community culture. You don't separate food and family. You're talking to a Southerner, and I really believe the South has it goin' on when it comes to food culture and passing recipes through the family. I grew up never eating out; my mom cooked, and my grandfather, Eugene, whom I named the restaurant after, was an outstanding cook. He made vinaigrette every night. He grew up on a farm in Tennessee. And so, you look at the traditions of foods in our South, and that becomes part of how we define ourselves as a family."

—Chef and restaurateur Linton Hopkins
on the culture of food

made from sheep's milk and goat's milk is easier to digest.

Peanut allergies in the United States are on the rise. Because of the severity of the allergic response in an individual with this allergy, parents are understandably concerned about the possibility of their child possessing it. For a long time, pediatricians recommended that infants should not be given peanuts until the age of two. New information suggests otherwise. Parents are left with no clear answers but are now advised to incorporate nuts in an infant's diet and not to wait. Knowing that children who are allergic usually react right away, I nervously gave Cody peanuts for the first time on a Monday morning when I knew

JOAN MCNAMARA founded and runs Joan's on Third, a culinary emporium that includes a much-loved cafe, marketplace, and full-service catering and event-planning company in Los Angeles. Her adult daughters, Carol and Susie, and Susie's husband, Chef Chester Hastings, all work with her. Susie and Chester have a son, Henry, who visits the store for a little bit every day. "I learned how to cook, I suppose, from my mother, the way you learn to walk or learn how to dance. I never took dancing lessons, you just did it, you know?" says McNamara. "When my children were born, I did the same thing with them. I have pictures of both girls standing on a chair—like my grandson now standing on a chair—stuffing the turkey for Thanksgiving. They'd wash their hands, and then I'd let them do it themselves. I always thought that letting them handle food was important, to just say 'look it, this is how you do this, now you do it.' I would watch, but they were allowed to do it themselves."

Joan McNamara and daughters Carol and Susie : MARY ANN MARINO

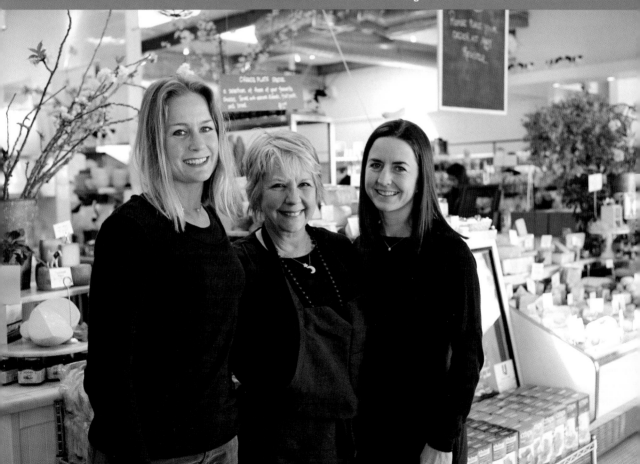

> "I started out with foods that might work together in terms of flavor and consistency, and I let my baby hold the food and play with it, smell it, and then taste it."
>
> —Alejandro Alcocer, New York City chef and epicurean

my pediatrician's office would be open. A new study indicates that peanut allergies may be treatable with a program of controlled peanut exposure that works similarly to a vaccine.

The Importance of Playing with Food

At six months, the age when most parents are just beginning to introduce solid food, an infant is captivated by touching and holding. He is fascinated by his food, and touching and playing with it is an important part of his development. Allowing him to play with his food creates a healthy curiosity and relationship with food. If your baby is reaching for your food, that's a good sign.

As babies grow, they often experience a surge in appetite. They begin to show independence and may want to feed themselves. This can and probably will be messy, so expect plenty of spills and splatters. If

TEACHING YOUR CHILD TO EAT

Teaching your child to eat is like teaching her anything else—it requires a lot of parenting. Here are some tips from chefs for feeding your young child:

- Take him shopping with you and talk to him, even when he is very young, about the foods you're cooking and eating. Even if he doesn't understand the content of what you are saying, you are building a foundation of communication and teaching about food.
- Let her watch you prepare her food. Even if she is not eating it, she will smell the aromas and be captivated by watching you mix and stir.
- Keep him with you when you're eating so he's exposed to the sights and smells of foods you enjoy.
- Acknowledge from the beginning that there will be challenges—some wasted food and some failures.

- Don't throw up your hands and give her the one or two things she'll readily eat. If you do, it'll become even harder for you to get her to try something new down the road. Instead, try to use encouragement and games to engage her.
- Build a repertoire of familiar foods and recipes that you're both happy with.
- Try to hold off on ready-made meals, fast foods, and sugars until he's older. (Sugars, including those in juice, have a profound effect on a child's brain, concentration, and energy level.) Let his palate develop with the flavor and nutrition of the real food you've made for him. It sets a precedent and a routine at the foundation of his understanding about what to eat.

•• Six months. **Your baby is entering a new world of flavor, texture, and color and is probably ready for solid food. She will revel in the way food feels in her hands, on her face, and—unfortunately!—the way it looks and sounds when it hits the floor. She loves manipulating objects, so let her play with a spoon and experiment with how it goes into the bowl. Make mealtimes part of her exploring time, reminding her to put the spoon in her mouth, too.**

•• Nine months. **At this stage, babies begin to show independence and want to feed themselves. This can be messy, but if you try to control your baby too much, he will sense your displeasure. Give him food that nurtures his curiosity and that he can handle by himself. Don't thwart his efforts or get into a struggle that could lead to a revolt even this early on; it's only a stage, and the pleasure he takes in messing with his food will subside. Expression is good! Touching and handling things is an indispensable preliminary to naming objects. Let him touch it all. His food and his plate and cup have different physical properties, and he will want to explore them.**

•• Twelve months. **By her first birthday, your child wants to explore her environment and test your reactions to it. She enjoys doing things herself, especially things she sees you do, so it's a good time to start tasting lots of different foods: Take a couple of bites yourself and offer her a bite to see what she thinks.**

At this age, a baby can hold a spoon by himself and drink from a cup. He begins to use a pincer grip. He likes to stack things, including food on his plate, and put things inside of other things, sorting them by color or shape. He can follow simple instructions like, "Hand me the napkin," and he understands *no*, but he may not listen.

•• Try to limit saying no. **The desire to look, touch, and feel is as urgent for your baby as hunger and as necessary for intellectual development as books will be later. You don't want her to lose her curiosity—you want to foster confidence. If your baby is reaching for your food, take that as a positive indicator of her developmental progress and encourage her exploration.**

you try to control your baby too much at this point, she will sense your displeasure and express frustration that she's not allowed to play. Give her food that nurtures her curiosity and that she can handle by herself.

Remember, these are developmental stages. The pleasure of messing with food will subside, and motor skills will improve. Right now, babies are starting to figure out how the world of objects works—they mush,

they fall, they bounce, they make patterns. Expression is good. This exposure to texture and color is the first step toward understanding objects.

Purees 101

Don't be intimidated by the idea of cooking for your growing baby. Even if you haven't had much experience in the kitchen, you can quickly learn your way

CYNTHIA EPPS is a metabolic nutritionist, board-certified lactation consultant, and infant-feeding specialist in private practice in Los Angeles. She trained at UCLA and the Cedars-Sinai Medical Center in Los Angeles. Her goal is teaching new mothers how to navigate their first year of motherhood.

MARCIA PELCHAT is a biopsychologist and associate member of the faculty at Monell Chemical Senses Center, a science institute in Philadelphia, where biologists, behavioral neuroscientists, ecologists, and chemists explore the science of our senses of taste and smell and how they relate to and affect human health.

around some basic techniques and ingredients. You will increase your confidence by handling these first simple purees.

There is a world of food out there just waiting to be pureed for your baby. Almost every fruit and vegetable can be pureed, thinned out if necessary, and served or frozen in batches and stored for up to six months. Fruits and vegetables can be enhanced with herbs and stocks and combined in flavorful ways, before or after freezing. Pureed food is both efficient and economical. Stored and/or frozen foods are especially handy when you need something fast, and stored favorites can be handy as a backup for meals that are not going over well.

It's a good idea to invest in durable, long-lasting kitchen equipment. A good food mill, for example, will last a lifetime and comes with multiple disks for versatility, whereas specialized cooking gear for infants may be made from plastic and may not be durable. Also, a pressure cooker can save time cooking dried grains and beans in bulk.

Purees can be smooth or a bit chunky. Make sure to remove all seeds. Seeds in fruits, when pureed, can be bitter, and some fruit seeds are not meant for consumption. Apples and pears and similar thin-skinned fruits need not be peeled if they are organic.

Most chefs' pantries are better stocked than most people's home pantries. The ingredients at their fingertips are often the best and freshest. Many times, they are exotic and expensive. While it may be impossible and impractical to replicate a restaurant pantry at home, it is certainly possible to stock your home pantry with different kinds of foods and rotate them to keep them fresh and seasonal.

Keep some ingredients ready to go so that you can concentrate more on the cooking and less on the prep work. Wash all your fruits and vegetables when you get them home from the market, before putting them away. Eric Bromberg, chef and cofounder of Blue Ribbon restaurants in and around the New York area, learned that he could make plain pasta in advance and refrigerate or even freeze it, then refresh it quickly by putting it back in boiling water for a minute or two. Buy cans of organic beans or cook a bag of dried beans to have around. Prepared beans and grains can be easily frozen, either in individual infant portions or family-size portions. Cover with a small amount of

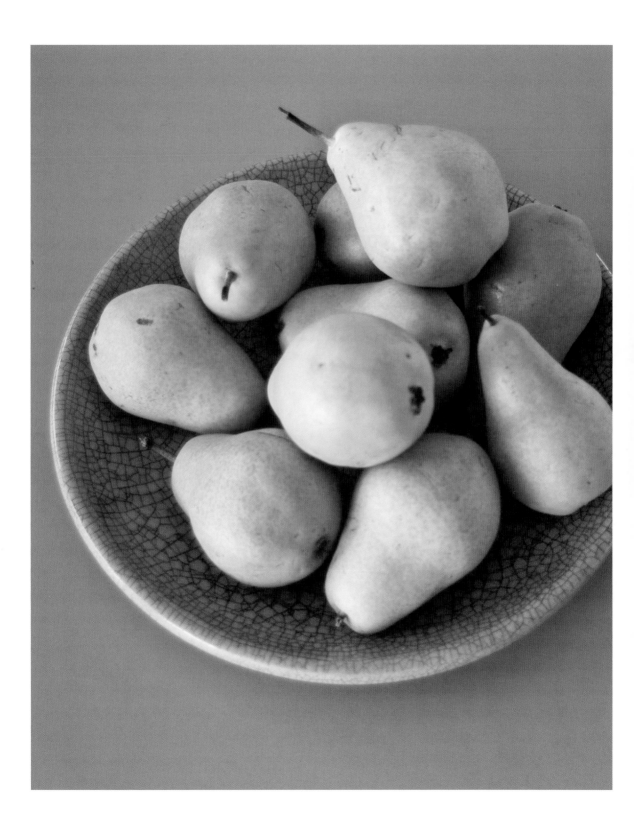

water or stock to prevent freezer burn. Most prepared and fresh foods can be frozen.

raw purees

Some fruits and vegetables, like bananas and avocados, can be pureed easily with a fork. With a basic food mill, you can puree any food that is a bit harder. I carried a small, simple hand-crank food mill with a travel pouch with me to make quick, easy baby meals from foods when we were out. Sometimes, I quickly grabbed frozen peas, lima beans, or fava beans to take with me and then pureed them as needed.

Here are some fresh foods that can be pureed easily: apricots, avocados, bananas, blueberries, cherries, fresh figs, kiwifruit, mangos, melons, nectarines, papayas, peaches, pears, thawed peas, strawberries (after baby's first birthday), watermelon.

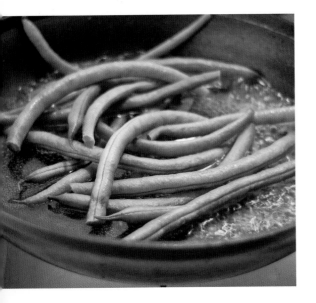

boiled purees

Sometimes I blanch long-cooking greens like kale until they are bright green and then take them out of the water to avoid overcooking them. All vegetables can be boiled, but boiling leaches flavor and nutrition out of the food and into the water, so use only a small amount of water or stock and incorporate the cooking liquid in the puree. After cooking, puree in a food processor or blender.

sautéed purees

Sautéing is the process of cooking foods in a pan with oil and/or butter. It's best to cook vegetables in small batches, not crowding the pan. At medium temperature they will brown, get a bit sweeter, and cook quickly in the oil and/or butter. Always use moderate temperatures when cooking with butter, as it can quickly burn (for higher heats with butter, coat the hot pan first with another oil like safflower before adding butter). Add water or broth to the pan after browning and cover with a lid for a minute or so to finish cooking the vegetables if needed. You can also cook them on a lower temperature to soften without browning to get a more delicate vegetable flavor. Herbs and other flavors like lemon can be quickly added at the end after you turn off the heat. Cut leafy vegetables into small pieces and cook for about five minutes. Harder vegetables, such as broccoli and potatoes, can be parboiled in advance. Fresh corn is succulent and sweet; you can simply cut it off the cob and sauté it in butter or oil. Greens like chard and spinach can be sautéed quickly in olive oil and make great purees.

For greens: Cut leafy pieces, discarding the stem, and wash but don't dry them. Add the greens dripping wet to a hot sauté pan with a bit of olive oil in it. Cook greens like spinach for only a few minutes; kale needs to be cooked for about seven to ten minutes. For longer cooking times, you can add a splash of water— or chicken or vegetable stock, for more flavor—to a pan that is getting dry. After cooking, puree in a food processor or blender.

For other vegetables: Cut into pieces and add to a hot pan with oil or melted butter. Stir every now and again to prevent sticking and to ensure the foods cook evenly. Cooking times will vary according to the freshness and kind of vegetable. Test for doneness with a fork. After cooking, puree in a food processor or blender with breast milk, water, or stock.

Vegetables that are delicious sautéed include asparagus, brussels sprouts, broccoli, carrots, cauliflower, corn, fresh fava beans, fennel, green beans, parsnips, potatoes, pumpkin, squashes, turnips, and zucchini.

steamed purees

It's easy to steam vegetables. By steaming instead of boiling, you avoid leaching any of the nutrients into the cooking water. The fruits and vegetables will have a cleaner and truer flavor. If you have a basket steamer, you can simply cut vegetables into small chunks and put them in the basket. Cook in a saucepan with an inch or two of water, with a lid on to keep the steam in. Cooking times vary; you can test for doneness with a fork. Vegetables are ready when they are still bright in color. If you don't have a

steamer, you can put the vegetable chunks in a sauté pan with a lid and a small amount of water. Add any herbs and spices just at the end. Incorporate the cooking water into your puree; it will be flavorful and nutritious. After cooking, puree vegetables in a food processor or blender.

Fruits and vegetables that taste great steamed include apples, asparagus, beets, broccoli, carrots, cauliflower, corn, green beans, parsnips, potatoes, pumpkin, squashes, turnips, and zucchini.

baked and roasted purees

The difference between baking and roasting is that baked foods are cooked without any oil. Both baking and roasting vegetables concentrate their flavor; roasting also makes vegetables sweeter. Both baking and roasting are fast, easy, and forgiving cooking methods.

To bake vegetables like beets and potatoes, wash and dry them and wrap them whole in aluminum foil or put them in a roasting dish and cover with a lid or foil. Foods can be baked or roasted whole or cut into chunks for quicker cooking. You can peel them or not. I put a variety of foods in the oven and cook them all at once—baking and roasting. It's a big time-saver.

Put your vegetables in a single layer, uncovered, in separate dishes (they may have different cooking times). To roast, drizzle a bit of olive or other oil over the pieces. (Fresh rosemary is a great addition to roasted vegetables. Mix it in with the oil.) Cooking times vary greatly. I bake beets and potatoes for about an hour at 400°F; smaller vegetables may require only fifteen or twenty minutes. Stir once or twice. After cooking and cooling, puree in a food processor or blender with breast milk, water, or stock.

Foods that are great baked or roasted include apricots, asparagus, beets, broccoli, brussels sprouts, carrots, cauliflower, eggplant, fennel, parsnips, peaches, peppers (green, red, and yellow), plums, potatoes (sweet and white), squashes (butternut and acorn), and turnips.

meat purees

Babies can start eating meat at seven to ten months of age, according to pediatricians, when they've mastered fruits and vegetables. Remember, though, that they don't have molars, so they can't chew pieces of meat the way they chew soft vegetables with their gums.

Any meat or meat dish can be pureed in a food processor. Try extra-small pieces of meatball or a sauce with finely ground meat.

Great First Baby Foods

Sweet potatoes can be cooked in advance and combined in many ways to explore flavors. They can be baked, boiled, steamed, or sautéed. Baking sweet potatoes concentrates their flavor and makes them sweeter.

Combine with: apple, pear, banana, chestnuts, leeks, persimmons, mushrooms, white beans, kale, or grains like oatmeal and brown rice.

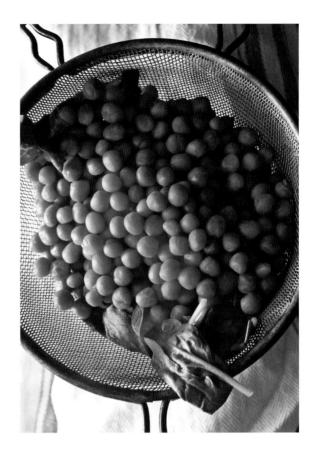

Thin out your puree with: orange juice, apple juice, lemon juice, or chicken or vegetable stock.

Add spices like: basil, cilantro, cloves, cinnamon, coriander, cumin, nutmeg, parsley, rosemary, sage, thyme, and garlic.

Peas are also easily combined with other foods. Peas overcook quickly, so boil, sauté, or steam them only briefly. If you are shelling fresh peas, you can make a pea broth from the pods and mix that in for deeper flavor. If the peas are frozen, you can simply defrost without cooking them.

Combine with: arugula, asparagus, carrots, celery, fava beans, leeks, potatoes, or spinach.

Thin out your puree with: carrot juice, lemon juice, chicken, or any other stock.

> **"I even season peas for Henry, my one-year-old grandson, because why not teach what is good flavor?"**
>
> —Joan McNamara, founder of Joan's on Third cafe and marketplace in Los Angeles

Add spices like: basil, chervil, cilantro, coriander, dill, mint, garlic, parsley, rosemary, sage, savory, tarragon, and thyme.

Bananas can be eaten and mashed raw and can also be baked and broiled.

Combine with: apricots, blueberries, cherries, coconut, guava, mangoes, oatmeal, papaya, raspberries, rice, strawberries, or sweet potatoes.

Thin out your puree with: coconut milk, lemon juice, or orange juice.

Add spices like: allspice, cardamom, cinnamon, cloves, and nutmeg.

Apples can easily be baked, sautéed, and stewed.

Combine with: apricots, blackberries, celery root, chestnuts, chicken, fennel, oatmeal, pears, plums, pork, prunes, pumpkin, rhubarb, rice, sweet potato.

Thin out your puree with: apple cider or juice, lemon juice, vegetable or chicken stock, or orange juice.

Add spices like: allspice, cardamom, cloves, coriander, cumin, or nutmeg.

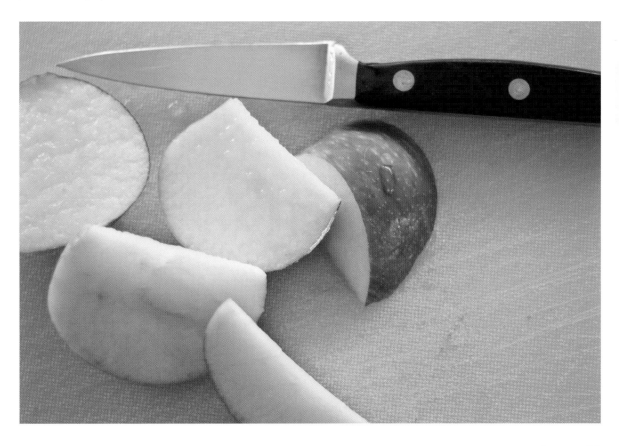

fresh pea and spinach puree

{ COLBY GARRELTS }

MAKES ABOUT 2 CUPS

Make this as a puree for infants, and for the adults, thin puree out with broth or water to make a soup. Add basil, mint, some pancetta, and for infants over one year old, swirl in some cream or top with feta cheese. This recipe works well with summer squash, too.

1 pound fresh or frozen peas
Handful fresh spinach
Reserved cooking water or broth for thinning
    as needed

1. If using fresh peas, shell the peas and steam them for 2 minutes in a steamer basket over boiling water until cooked through and bright green. If using frozen peas, quickly blanch them in a bit of boiling water. Reserve any leftover cooking water to use for thinning out the puree.

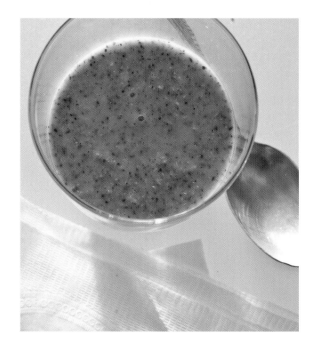

2. Puree the peas and the handful of fresh spinach in a blender in batches at high speed. (*Note:* Be cautious about blending hot ingredients in your blender, as this has a tendency to force the top off midblend, splattering the blender contents. Don't fill your blender canister more than half full, and hold the lid down with a folded dish towel while you're operating the blender.) Add the reserved water as necessary to achieve a smooth, thin consistency. You may wish to push the puree through a sieve to get rid of any remaining skins.

3. Cool and store in the fridge for up to 5 days or freeze in ice cube trays.

wild greens puree

{ DIANE FORLEY }

MAKES ABOUT 3 CUPS

Make this as a puree for infants and thin with breast milk, formula, brown rice cereal, stock, or some mashed potato. For older children and adults, the puree can be combined with broth, noodles, and chicken and made into a soup, thinned and made into a sauce and served over noodles, or used to make Poached Chicken with Wild Greens (page 29).

2 cups chopped kale

2 cups chopped collard greens

2 tablespoons olive oil

1 teaspoon salt

1 cup plus 2 tablespoons water, divided

½ cup fresh flat-leaf parsley leaves

¼ cup fresh basil leaves

2 cups chopped spinach

Breast milk, formula, rice cereal, stock, or cooked white potato as needed for thinning

1. Add kale and collard greens into a saucepan with olive oil, salt, and 2 tablespoons water. Cover with lid and let steam over medium heat, stirring occasionally, until greens turn bright and soften, about 10 minutes.

2. Add parsley, basil, and spinach and cook 5 more minutes to wilt spinach and herbs.

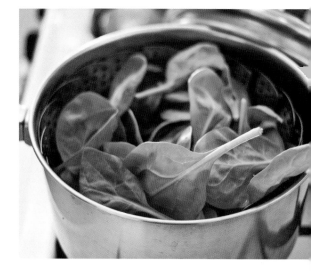

3. Let cool. Transfer to a blender and puree with the remaining cup of water.

4. Serve thinned with breast milk, formula, rice cereal, stock, or cooked white potato as needed, and portion remainder into ½-cup servings and freeze in resealable plastic bags.

millet cauliflower puree

{ PETER BERLEY }

SERVES 4

Make this as a puree for infants, but for toddlers it can be mashed instead. Add the crispy caramelized onions for older children and adults.

Millet Cauliflower Puree:

1 small head cauliflower, cored and roughly chopped
   (about 3 cups)

1 cup millet, washed and drained

½ teaspoon salt

3 cups water

Crispy Caramelized Onions:

1 cup olive oil

2 medium onions, very thinly sliced into crescents

For Millet Cauliflower Puree:

1. Combine the cauliflower, millet, salt, and water in a heavy saucepan.

2. Bring to a boil over high heat.

3. Reduce the heat to low and simmer, covered, for 25 to 30 minutes, until the water has been absorbed.

4. Mash the millet and cauliflower until smooth.

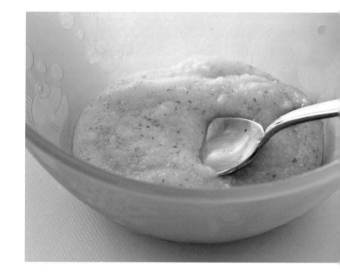

For Crispy Caramelized Onions:

1. Heat the oil in a wide sauté pan over medium heat.

2. Add the onions and sauté slowly for 20 to 30 minutes, until the onions are a deep golden brown.

3. Regulate the heat to prevent burning. Stir often for even browning.

4. Drain the onions and reserve the oil.

5. To serve, drizzle a bit of the oil over the mash and top with a mound of crispy onions.

wild greens soup with noodles

{ DIANE FORLEY }

Noodles with soup is a fast and easy standard in our house—a big dollop of greens puree mixed in the soup adds a big nutritious boost and a subtle earthy flavor. Sometimes we add delicate slices of poached chicken (page 29).

2 cups Wild Greens Puree, more or less to your liking (page 21)
4 cups chicken broth
1 package ramen, soba, or udon noodles, cooked according to package directions (break into small pieces for infants first)
1 tablespoon butter (optional)
Sprinkle of Parmesan cheese

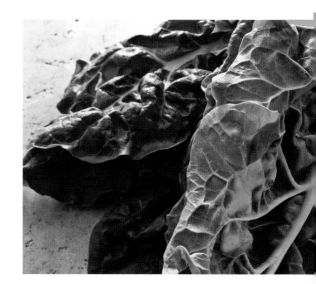

1. Combine puree with chicken broth in a saucepan and bring to a simmer.

2. Add cooked ramen noodles to warm broth mixture.

3. Finish with butter and sprinkle with Parmesan cheese.

pumpkin soup with coconut, peanuts, and scallions

{ B. T. NGUYEN }

SERVES 4

Pumpkins are not just for jack-o'-lanterns and pies. Good choices for cooking are sugar pumpkins and heirloom varieties such as the gray-skinned Jarrahdale, the white-skinned Cucurbita, or a delicious cheese pumpkin that has a pale orange skin. When selecting a pumpkin, remember that a fresh pumpkin or squash will be a lot easier to peel and more flavorful than one that's been on the shelves for a while.

Cody and I play guessing games when cutting up fruits and squashes about what color the insides will be. This is a warm, comforting soup and the peanut and scallion garnish livens it up for older children and adults and adds a welcome and surprising crunch. Use less broth or water to make a thicker puree that is more like baby food.

4 cups vegetable or chicken broth
3 cups pumpkin (½ small pumpkin—approximately 2
    pounds) or butternut squash, peeled and cut into
    2-inch cubes
⅓ cup sliced galangal (see note at right)
8 ounces coconut milk
2 tablespoons soy sauce, Maggi or other quality brand
1½ teaspoons raw or other sugar
1½ teaspoons sea salt
¼ cup roasted peanuts, finely chopped or crushed
3 scallions, white and light green parts only,
    chopped fine

1. In a medium saucepan over medium heat bring broth to a boil.

2. Add pumpkin and galangal (in cheesecloth to remove quickly and easily; see note below) and simmer over medium heat for 25 minutes or until the pumpkin is soft (fresher pumpkins will cook faster).

3. Turn heat down and add coconut milk, soy sauce, raw sugar, and salt and stir until combined and sugar is dissolved. Turn the heat off and let cool; remove the galangal.

4. Puree for babies and freeze leftovers. For adults and older babies, serve with finely chopped roasted peanuts and scallions sprinkled on top.

Notes: Galangal is a mild type of ginger. It has a floral aroma and is a bit tougher to cut than ginger. Try going to an Asian market to find it. Some people recommend substituting ginger, but ginger at the same quantities is too pungent. You can make the soup using ginger sparingly or make the soup without it. Using butternut squash will make the soup sweeter than using pumpkin.

Wrapping spices and herbs in cheesecloth is a great way to give flavor to soups and a pot of beans and is easy to remove when the cooking is finished. Another great trick is to put them in a refillable tea bag. Try it here with the galangal, which is a bit too fibrous to puree with the soup and is better removed after cooking.

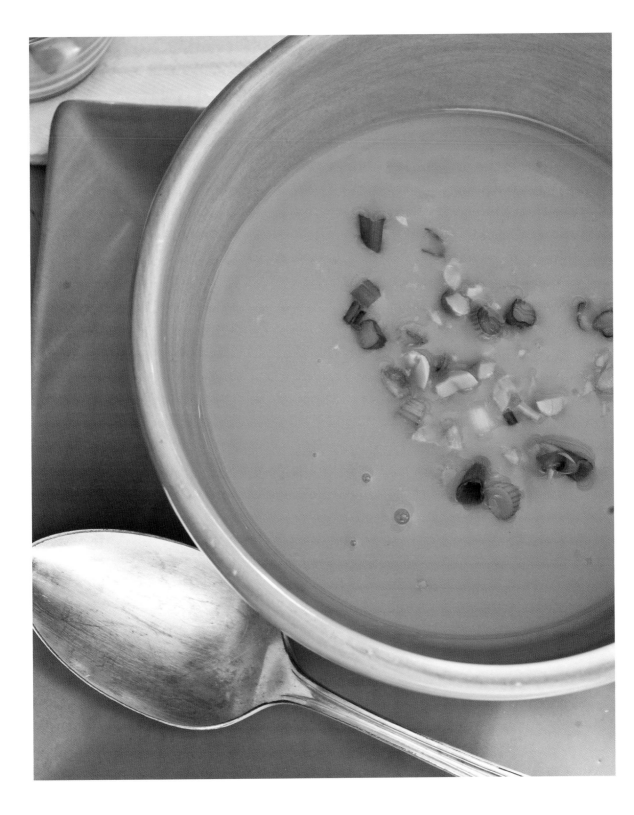

cannellini bean dip

{ PIERO SELVAGGIO }

MAKES ABOUT 2 CUPS

"I was amazed," says Chef Piero Selvaggio of his daughter dipping bread into a cannellini bean dip one night out for dinner. "Sasha, who is ten months old, devoured the first little morsel, the second little morsel, and I thought, 'It makes so much sense—it's simple and so flavorful and it's good—and it's healthy.'" Selvaggio says this dip is similar to hummus, but the use of cannellini beans, popular in Italy, makes it Italian in spirit. You can use dried beans cooked with rosemary and other herbs for a richer flavor. Serve pureed beans with a poached egg nestled on top for a complete meal or as a dollop atop Diane Forley's Ratatouille with Balsamic Vinegar, Honey, and Basil (page 55). Use the best-quality fruity extra-virgin olive oil you can to drizzle over the dip.

1 can cannellini beans or white kidney beans, drained and rinsed

1½ teaspoons white wine vinegar

1 clove garlic, chopped

1½ teaspoons Worcestershire sauce

Kosher salt to taste

Pinch black pepper

¼ cup good olive oil

1 tablespoon chopped chives

Italian bread or other bread, or breadsticks warmed for serving

Cucumber sliced into sticks

Carrot sticks

1. In a food processor puree the beans with the white wine vinegar, garlic, Worcestershire sauce, and salt and pepper. Gradually add the olive oil with the machine running and puree until smooth.

2. Serve the dip in a bowl with chives sprinkled over the top and with warmed Italian bread or breadsticks, cucumber, and carrot sticks.

scrambled eggs and kale

{ PIERO SELVAGGIO }

SERVES 4

Piero Selvaggio says that kids love egg whites, so he adds more whites than yolks when making scrambled eggs. Kale can have a strong flavor, and sometimes we add a small bunch of fresh basil that Cody likes. If you are holding off on serving dairy, you can make this without the cheese. Serve with toast, fresh berries, and a side of yogurt.

2 large eggs

5 egg whites

1 teaspoon olive oil

6 ounces kale (cavolo nero preferred), parboiled and
   finely chopped

2 ounces fresh mushrooms, sliced

4 ounces mozzarella cheese, shredded or chopped
   if fresh

Sea salt

Black pepper, optional

1. In a bowl, mix the eggs and egg whites with a splash of water to combine.

2. Heat the olive oil in a nonstick pan over medium heat. Add the eggs and cook, stirring, until the eggs come together. Add the kale, mushrooms, and mozzarella. Stir together and cook just until the cheese melts. Sprinkle with salt and pepper and serve.

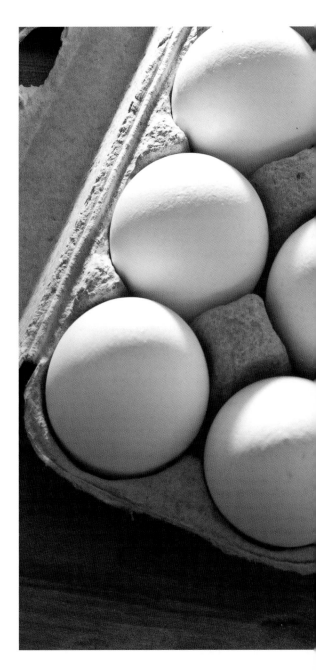

roast chicken with potatoes and kale

{ PIERO SELVAGGIO }

SERVES 4

I was always looking for ways to incorporate greens like kale into meals for Cody because they are so rich in nutrients. I love the flavor of kale when it's cooked right, but its earthy flavor can make it a tricky addition to dishes. While kale is sweeter in the wintertime, it is available year-round at markets. I like using the kale that has long, thin, dark blue green leaves, called Lacinato or dinosaur kale. If your child has never had kale before, start with adding a bit less to the recipe. If you are preparing this for infants or babies still learning to chew or unfamiliar with meat, chop chicken into very small cubes and make sure not to overcook, because the meat will be too chewy and dry. Kale and squash are a wonderful combination, and you can substitute any winter squash for the potatoes. To puree, remove the chicken from the bone and puree with the vegetables and a bit of chicken stock.

½ pound fresh kale, washed, stems removed, and chopped
½ pound small potatoes (or winter squash like butternut or acorn), chopped
1 onion, chopped
2 tablespoons olive oil
Sea salt and fresh pepper
3 chicken legs
Pinch of paprika
½ lemon, juiced

1. Preheat the oven to 450°F.

2. Spread kale, potatoes (or squash), and onion onto a large pan. Drizzle the oil over the vegetables, sprinkle with salt and pepper, and mix to evenly coat the vegetables. Cut the chicken legs halfway through at the joint between the thigh and drumstick. Rub salt and pepper and paprika all over the chicken and set atop the vegetables. Cover the pan with foil and bake for 20 minutes.

3. Remove the foil and continue to bake for another 20 minutes or until the chicken is cooked through and tender. Cut the chicken into small pieces for infants who can chew and add a squeeze of lemon. Serve alongside the vegetables.

poached chicken with wild greens

{ DIANE FORLEY }

When poached chicken is cooked right, it has an incredible and lovely silky texture, perfect for infants first learning to eat meat. But if the chicken is just a bit overcooked, it will get rubbery. One way to save time in the kitchen on busy days is to have poached chicken ready in the fridge to dice up for an older baby's snack or to add to soup, or for older kids and adults to make chicken salad or sliced chicken sandwiches. Use this chicken in Diane Forley's recipe for Wild Greens Soup with Noodles (page 23).

2 boneless, skinless chicken breasts
Broth or water to cover
Salt and pepper
1 cup Wild Greens Puree (page 21)

1. Clean and dry the chicken breasts.

2. Pound the chicken breasts so that they have an even thickness throughout and are no more than ½-inch thick, for even cooking.

3. Put enough broth (makes the chicken more flavorful) or water to cover the chicken breasts in a saucepan and heat to a low simmer.

4. Add chicken breasts and poach over low heat, skimming off and discarding any foam. Poach chicken until just cooked through, about 5 minutes. Watch the chicken carefully so as not to overcook.

5. Remove chicken to a cutting board and reserve the broth to thin the puree or for another use. Season the chicken with salt and pepper to taste and let rest for a couple of minutes.

6. Warm Wild Greens Puree in a pan over low heat, adding broth as needed to thin.

7. Slice the chicken and serve topped with warmed puree.

lemongrass chicken curry

{ B. T. NGUYEN }

SERVES 4

Curry is a traditional Vietnamese comfort food. This is not an actual curry; it is more like a stew. The dish can be pureed and thinned with broth or breast milk if necessary or pureed with plain cooked rice or potatoes. When cooking, the chili powder should be put in toward the end of cooking, after the baby's portion is removed. I like prepping everything the night before so it is ready. Chef B. T. Nguyen recommends serving the curry soupy with freshly baked French bread. I often entice Cody to taste things by first dipping in some bread.

Marinade:

¼ lemongrass stalk, tough outer leaves removed and stalk chopped

1 shallot, chopped

2 cloves garlic, chopped

1 teaspoon chopped galangal or ginger (use less for infants) (see note on page 24)

1½ teaspoons chopped fresh cilantro

2 tablespoons coconut milk

1 tablespoon chopped fresh basil

2 green onions, white parts only, sliced (reserve green parts for curry)

1 tablespoon lime juice

Curry:

2 boneless, skinless chicken breasts, cubed

¼ cup vegetable oil, divided

1 pound potatoes (or batata), peeled and evenly chopped

½ onion, chopped small

2 medium carrots, peeled and evenly chopped

½ cup chicken stock or coconut water

7 ounces coconut milk (about half a can)

¾ stalk lemongrass, tough outer leaves removed and stalk pounded to crush and soften

1 teaspoon best-quality fish sauce

1 teaspoon palm sugar or golden granulated sugar

Salt and pepper

½ teaspoon chili powder (eschew for infants, adjust for children)

Small bunch cilantro

Small bunch basil

2 green onions, green parts only, sliced

For the Marinade:

Grind the lemongrass in a spice or coffee grinder. Add the rest of the marinade ingredients and process until smooth. Rub onto the chicken cubes, massaging a bit to coat evenly. Marinate covered and refrigerated overnight or at least 3 hours. Remove from the refrigerator an hour before cooking.

For the Curry:

1. Heat 2 tablespoons of oil in heavy-bottomed pan over medium heat. Add potatoes, onion, and carrots and cook, stirring occasionally, until evenly browned, about 5 minutes. Transfer browned vegetables to a plate.

2. In the same pan heat the remaining 2 tablespoons oil and add marinated chicken. Cook to brown for 5 minutes, turning occasionally to brown on all sides.

3. Add stock or coconut water, coconut milk, and crushed lemongrass stalks and return the potatoes and carrots back to the pan. Mix well and bring to boil.

4. Add fish sauce, sugar, salt and pepper, and chili powder (if using); simmer on low heat for 35 to 40 minutes, or until potatoes are soft.

5. Portion onto plates and sprinkle cilantro leaves, chopped basil, and green onion on top to serve.

Note: Lemongrass stalks have a lovely elusive flavor but are fibrous and can be hard to prepare correctly, especially for young children. It works best to cut the yellow section of stalk into thin slices and grind them in a mini grinder/chopper or food processor that handles small quantities, adding a bit of water or oil if necessary. For very small amounts pound them into a paste with a mortar and pestle.

after purees

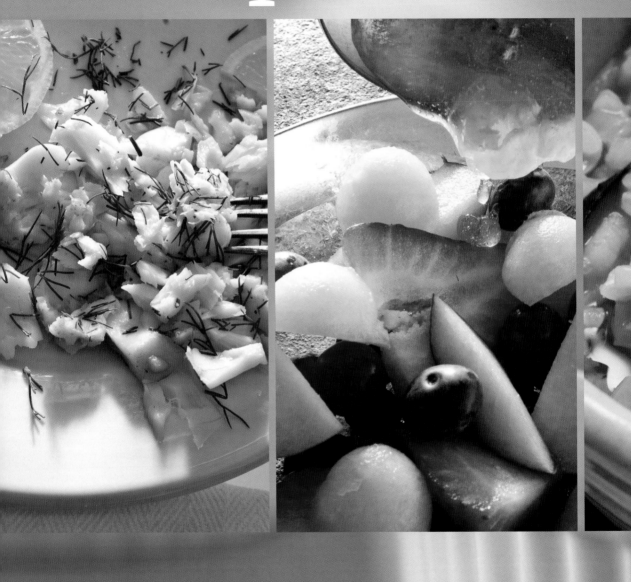

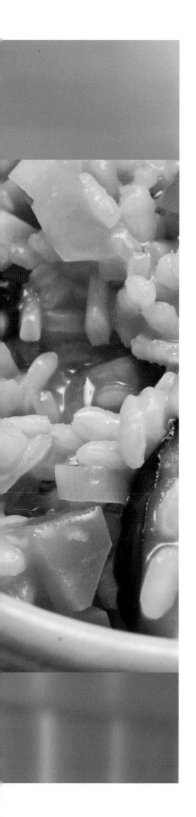

THE BEGINNING OF ADVENTUROUS EATING

ages one to two-and-a-half

It's true toddlers are fun and silly. They are experimenting and learning new things constantly. Chefs tap into and embrace their curious nature in the way they feed their children at this age by enthusiastically introducing them to the whole world of food, its wondrous colors and shapes and interesting flavors and textures. There's almost nothing a toddler can't eat, and chefs don't hold back, offering them tastes of everything in the pantry, on the stove, or in the market.

Bring Them to the Table

While many parents slip into a routine of feeding toddlers separate meals of bland foods like pasta with butter, chefs bring their children to the table with them, introducing them early on to foods with the complex textures and flavors that they themselves enjoy. "Our kids went right from eating purees to eating what we were eating," says Eric Bromberg, chef and cofounder of Blue Ribbon restaurants in New York City.

Alejandro Alcocer, epicurean and founder of Green Brown Orange (Green Catering, Brown Café, and Orange Épicerie) in New York City, rattles off a list of the unusual things he feeds his toddler, Joaquin: "Shrimp, lobster, asparagus, and oysters. He eats what we're eating. We sit down together and cut what we're eating into small pieces, and he eats with his hands." Feeding children expensive and exotic ingredients is not necessary, but feeding them a wide variety of foods is. At this age it's important to make sure they are learning to like the flavors of healthy foods, including vegetables and whole grains, and are learning to like the experience of eating foods with new flavors—both of which can be tricky.

repeatedly offer a variety of flavors

Toddlers, like babies, have an abundance of taste buds that are spread around their mouths, including on the inner surfaces of their cheeks. They have an amazing ability to decipher flavors. Cutting-edge science at the Monell Chemical Research lab helps us to understand that all babies are born with a preference for sweet flavors and can distinguish between different types of sweet foods. A taste for bitter flavors—like the flavors of some vegetables—is learned. Children

"Cooking . . . I find that it's a good time to spend with your kid. . . . We got Zen a play kitchen, and every morning she's like, 'What do you want for breakfast, Daddy?' We got to the point where as long as I don't have to get to work super early, she'll want to make me breakfast. . . . It's becoming really fun; I always show her that, too. You've got to make it fun. I don't want to be serious all the time. I certainly don't want to be serious with a two-year-old . . . I just think you have to make it a fun experience for the kids. If you don't, you're kind of missing out."

—Zack Gross, chef and owner of Z Grille in St. Petersburg, Florida

grow to like foods by eating them repeatedly. Studies show that toddlers who are given lots of different vegetables do learn to enjoy them, and those children also end up liking vegetables they haven't previously tasted more often. Science suggests that children have a critical learning window—from when they begin eating solid foods until about two years old—to adjust to eating a wide variety of foods.

Chefs teach their children early on to enjoy a variety of flavors by repeatedly offering them a diverse selection of foods and foods that have unique flavor characteristics—earthiness, richness, bitterness, pungency, and sourness.

"One of the things that we continuously do is just keep introducing things to Madi. When Meg's parents were down here for New Year's—when she was about a year and a half old—I shoved a spoonful of caviar in Madi's mouth. She chomped it down and ate it. A lot of times kids don't like certain things because they are too strongly flavored and they like more sweet

and mild food, but for Madi, I just go full bore on it," says Colby Garrelts, chef and co-owner with his wife, Megan, of Bluestem restaurant in Kansas City.

Chefs agree that learning to eat a variety of foods as a toddler is critical to eating and enjoying a broad range of foods later on. "Bring your kids into the lives you lead," Marc Murphy, owner and executive chef of Benchmarc restaurants in New York recommends. "We just cut up whatever we are eating into small enough pieces so they don't choke. Whatever we make is what they'll eat."

"Babies can taste so many different flavor profiles," says B. T. Nguyen, Tampa chef and restaurateur. "So let them eat what you eat. They will open up to it. But if you say 'my kids only eat chicken,' you know what, you are not opening them up to let them experience other flavors."

take your kids to a farmers' market

Diane Forley, chef and co-owner with her chef husband, Michael Otsuka, of Flourish Bakery in Scarsdale, New York, says that her daughter, Olivia, can identify a lot of foods and ingredients from having shopped with her at an early age at the farmers' market and the grocery store: "She can identify arugula."

Alcocer describes going to farms and introducing his sons to "the whole process. I've gotten involved with some local farmers, and worked with them to learn about organic farming. Through visiting these people, Constantin is able to appreciate and understand where food comes from." He also talks about taking Constantin to Africa, where "we see people prepare food with a fire in a hut. He sees that people can

"Introduce as many new things as possible without overwhelming the child. I think children can very easily get overwhelmed with flavors and tastes."

—Cathal Armstrong, chef and co-owner of Restaurant Eve; Eamonn's, a Dublin Chipper; and The Majestic in Alexandria, Virginia

gather foods and just eat them. He sees that they have no access to sugar and processed foods. He knows that there are people in the world who don't have so many choices."

don't emphasize your own food dislikes
Chefs also agree that it's important not to convey your own distaste for certain foods to your children. "Don't ever say you don't like something in front of your kid," Murphy advises. "It will influence them. They either won't like the thing you say you don't like, or they'll use it as an opportunity to create their own dislikes." Frank Proto, executive chef with Murphy of Benchmarc restaurants in New York, says, "My wife doesn't like peas, but she doesn't say so in front of the kids."

establish your own mealtime routines
Though many chefs' schedules make it difficult for them to have regular meals with their children, they acknowledge that it does make a difference to sit down to a meal together. Cathal Armstrong, chef and co-owner of Restaurant Eve; Eamonn's, a Dublin Chipper; and The Majestic in Alexandria, Virginia, says that his children's eating suffered during a time when both he and his wife, Michelle, were working long hours and not able to eat dinner together with their children. Because chefs typically work during dinner hours and on weekends, many devote time in the morning to cook breakfast together with their children.

Children at this age love familiarity and routines. They begin to make associations between foods and experiences. Zack Gross, chef at Z Grille at St. Petersburg, Florida, reminisces about how his mom cooked tacos when he was a child or made "amazing" French toast for him. "I loved the way she made it and loved her for making it." While Gross admits it's not the healthiest snack food, he relishes eating cotton candy at the baseball game with his daughter, Zen.

Cook Well and Give Kids Options
Armstrong explains that cooking well is important for children because "if the food tastes good, they are much more likely to eat it. I do think being a good cook is an important part of introducing food to children, especially when you want to introduce challenging foods like brussels sprouts instead of carrots. Carrots are easy because they are sweet. Brussels sprouts are a much more difficult challenge. It's just a matter of getting them to try a little bit; try a quarter and chances are they are going to hate it the first couple of times. Seasoning, too, is an important part of food," adds Armstrong. "Cooking things they recognize and want to eat is also important."

"Giving kids a choice and not always deciding everything for them—especially at two, when they go through that independent phase—is important; they can be really cranky during the terrible twos. I think allowing them those independent choices even at a young age is crucial," says Armstrong. "Food is one of the ways you can do that," adds Megan Garrelts. "They eat what they like from what

ZACK GROSS AND HIS WIFE, JEN, have a busy urban restaurant, Z Grille, in St. Petersburg, Florida, that is both elegant and edgy. It serves adventurous, casual-yet-gourmet fare that is both playful and decadent, like his Dr Pepper–fried Ribs or his Cornflake Sage Fried Chicken served with a bacon waffle. In 2009, he was nominated for the James Beard Award as Best Chef in the South. They have a daughter, Zen. Zack says, "I like to go home and make a nice piece of chicken with some cooked rice with gravy—something that's very comforting—that's what I like to eat at home.... I want to spend time with my kid and I want to get her to eat and make sure she enjoys eating and gets pleasure out of it. Cooking with her is getting her to enjoy it more. I find that it's a good time to spend with your kid, too. My mom taught me how to cook."

Chef Zack Gross and daughter Zen : JEN GROSS

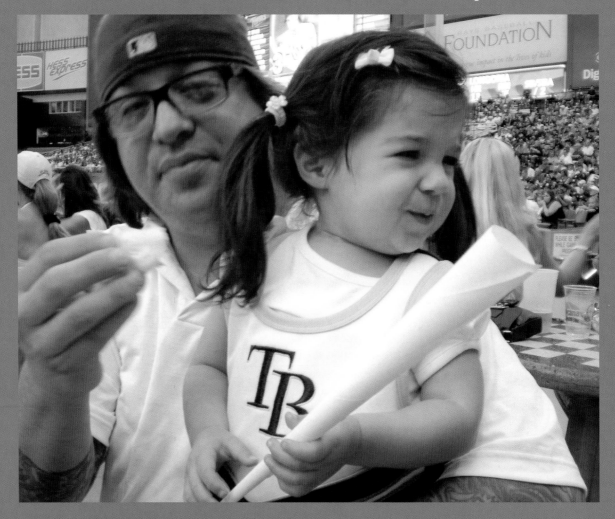

we cook and we don't force them to eat what they don't like," says Murphy.

"I'll give her a choice, like, 'You can have one of these three things.' She's at an age where she can choose," says Ana Sortun. "For lunch today, I asked her if she wanted a ham sandwich or a hot dog or whatever. She'll tell me what she wants. We'll do the same thing for breakfast. 'Do you want oatmeal, do you want cold cereal, or do you want eggs?' She loves eggs and waffles. Sometimes she'll want that, and sometimes she'll choose oatmeal."

Cooking braises, and more forgiving stews, is an easy way to make flavorful food for a toddler. "I definitely go traditional at home. I roast chicken and make corn on the cob and grill steaks, but in the winter when we are not outside as much, we'll braise lamb and roast some root vegetables and things like that," says Colby Garrelts.

I took Colby's suggestions and often made braises and stews for our family's dinner when Cody was at this age. The meat was easy to chew and flavorful. I made short ribs and lots of tender roasted meats like pork tenderloin. Since Cody napped best at home, I would take advantage of this and start a dish while he was napping in the middle of the day. I'd brown the meat and add onions and other vegetables, broth, and wine and then let it cook slowly. I liked that we had something already prepared to come home to and could avoid a hectic rush to make dinner. And I liked that the house always had the delicious aromas of slow-cooked foods. I'd open the lid so Cody could peek at what was cooking, and as a bonus, there would usually be enough to freeze some for a future meal.

Some dishes were too much for Cody. I would try to modify the stronger flavors of these by adding cheese, cream, or butter or adding a starch like potatoes. Many modern chefs use herbs and lemon to brighten and crisp the flavors of dishes. "You know little kids, they can't take a lot of spices and flavorings—they like it simple," says Peter Berley. "Sometimes I'll make a kid version of what we're eating that's a bit simpler than ours," says Forley. "But if we're having something we know they'll like—for instance, baked chicken—then I won't adjust the menu for the kids; we'll just all eat the same thing." With kids, it's about finding the right balance between introducing new flavors and foods and adjusting those recipes that may still be a bit overwhelming for them.

Enjoy Eating and Cooking with Your Kids

It's fun to be silly with a toddler, and eating with your toddler should be enjoyable. "I love food. That's why I do what I do, so I don't want to come home and eat boring food," says Colby Garrelts. I agree, and I wanted Cody to eat well so we could enjoy meals together. I liked making special things for us to eat and enjoy as a family.

Lure children into eating by setting an example and enjoying food yourself, and by having them participate and play in the kitchen. Keeping your kids in the kitchen with you is important at this age. Not only are they continuing to become familiar with the sights and smells of all the foods you are cooking, but they are naturally curious and will want to watch you at work. They will want to imitate you, and giving them

> "I've moved my cutting board out of the normal spot where it was, over by the sink, and I've created a little square over by the stove.... Zen can watch everything. I put the *mise en place* in front of her and then she can dump it in the pan, or I help her do it. 'Oh, I cooked it!' she'll say. And she has more of an appreciation to eat things."
>
> —Zack Gross, chef at Z Grille in St. Petersburg, Florida

some tools to play with will make them feel like they are involved. Cody played intently with the salad spinner, a bag of beans, and a wooden spoon while in the kitchen with me. Every now and again he'd pop up to help mix something, and then he'd go back to playing. Sometimes he pretends he's cooking pasta in a little pan that I give him, and he asks me to taste it.

Sally Kravich, a natural health expert, says, "What we feed our kids is so important. And so is their connectedness to it. That's why I teach kids about planting seeds and letting them grow. They get connected to the plant itself. It's why I always had them make messes and play in the kitchen, putting their hands in it and creating lots of different things, because then they are a part of it. Saying, 'Taste this, taste that. Let's see what this thing tastes like.'"

Cody and I planted a simple herb garden together so we could both dig in the dirt and take care of something and watch it grow. Planting our garden gave us an opportunity to smell, taste, and identify herbs. We would go out together and pinch off some basil or parsley. Having the experience of growing and picking the herbs helped Cody like those flavors. Sortun gets most of her produce from her husband's farm, Siena Farms. Siena, their daughter, spends a lot of time

there. "She likes watermelon radishes and arugula. She knows where they come from. That's a big part of it," says Sortun. Sortun organizes field trips for Siena's school, and she realized that kids would eat and enjoy foods growing at the farm that their parents swore they wouldn't eat at home.

Picky Eaters

While toddlers will fully join in and eat all the interesting foods you eat, quirky food phases and picky eating also begin for lots of kids at this age. Colby Garrelts says of his daughter, Madi, "She's not always a real good eater, and it seems like she's been going through different cycles or times when she'll eat better than others." Quirky eaters might relish a food one day and completely refuse it the next, ask enthusiastically for something and then play with it but not eat it. They may eat only tiny portions or not eat at all. Trying to reason with any toddler doesn't work particularly well, but distraction and silliness are good strategies to get them eating and enjoying their food. Toddlers sense what's important to you; they will follow your lead because they want to keep you happy. "The first time we gave Eve potatoes she spat them out," says Armstrong. "And then I gave her a little bit and I said, 'Don't spit it out.' Then I gave her a little more, and now she's older and she says, 'Please can I have some mashed potatoes for dinner?'"

Picky eating is very common among toddlers. Some picky eaters may be born that way. Scientists have found that the ability to taste may be genetically related to the number of taste buds on a person's tongue. While adults have six thousand taste buds, babies have up to ten thousand. The so-called genetic "supertaster" is not necessarily a picky eater and vice versa. He may have as many as eleven hundred taste buds per square centimeter of tongue compared to as few as eleven taste buds in the same size area, creating a vastly different experience and response to flavors like sweetness and bitterness. "Sweet and sour are two tastes that kids do like as they are developing," says Berley, "but things like spicy and bitter, more complex flavors, really develop much, much later for the taste buds."

"Spicy food is hot, and it hurts to eat it," adds Otsuka. "Kids probably don't have the ability to discern that pain from any other pain. They are still developing. And any kind of pain is bad from a kid's perspective." In fact most children even from cultures known for their spicy cuisine dislike the burning sensation from eating spicy foods. Science shows that the brain actually thinks the tongue is on fire, and even adults who enjoy eating spicy foods experience them as painful. While there is no correlation between age and tolerance for spicy foods, finding spicy foods palatable is learned, and at some point it just clicks that feeling that the burn on the tongue is stimulating and pleasurable.

All foods can be sweetened a bit without adding sugars. Roasted meats can be cooked with red onions that add sweetness or they can be served with gravies or fruit sauces and relishes. Vegetables can be roasted to caramelize their natural sugars and make them sweeter. Vegetables like carrots and corn are sweet on their own. Alternatively, some vegetables can be baked or served in a cheese sauce, which usually goes over well with kids.

Although Cody was never a truly fussy eater, he did have picky phases that were both surprising and frustrating. It's hard to be motivated to cook for a picky eater, and sometimes it's best to keep things simple. There were times when I resorted to easy favorites at home for dinner, like nachos made with black beans with some Greek yogurt for dipping and some avocado on the side. Cody always enjoys these nachos, and I knew overall it was a pretty healthy dinner.

Children can become fussy eaters for a number of reasons. They may develop sensitivities to certain tastes, smells, or textures, or they may be imitating parents' fussy eating habits. There is "a family resemblance in broad attitudes in things like food neophobia—fear of trying new foods," explains Marcia Pelchat, a biopsychologist. "So if you have parents who are suspicious of food, worried about food, with a lot of anxiety about food, you are going to notice that also in their children." Fussy eating habits are also more likely to develop when parents punish or reward their children's eating behaviors.

Chefs' children are no exception, and chefs agree that it's important to keep trying, even when your child refuses a food. Some children need more time to get used to the various textures, colors, and tastes of new foods. The biggest challenge with feeding young kids—especially picky ones—is novel foods and new flavors. Studies show that approximately one quarter of parents with infants and toddlers think their children dislike a food after serving it only twice. "When I introduce a food to my one-year-old and he doesn't like it, I

> "They love broccoli, then all of a sudden they don't like broccoli anymore. It's just phases. Like anything else with raising kids, it's a full-time job. You have to keep at it. You can't slack off. Otherwise they develop those bad habits. It's your job—it's your duty."
>
> —Andrea Curto-Randazzo, Miami chef

keep trying, even in the same meal," says Susie, Los Angeles cafe and marketplace owner Joan McNamara's daughter. Chefs emphasize that it's important to "go with the flow" and rely on what's working at any given time, without discontinuing the process of trying new foods. Studies show that children who do dislike a particular food or ingredient at this age will accept and enjoy that food after repeated exposure. In other words, for most of us, enjoying the flavors of a variety of foods is learned, and it requires patient conditioning to teach toddlers to like those foods, too.

Forley says, "It's a daily investigation between parents and kids. There are no hard-and-fast rules. My daughter, Olivia, used to like certain things, and now she's gone off them. Maybe her taste for the things she is rejecting will come back, but for now we have to work with what she'll do and what she won't." Still, it's important not to give in to a toddler's preference for an overly simplified and limited diet.

Keep in mind that children at this age probably won't remember a food they've eaten from one sitting to the next. They will certainly recognize distinct foods with colors and shapes that appeal to them, but most children will not immediately remember foods they've disliked. Gross says of his daughter, Zen, "When she doesn't want it, she says 'no, please'—she's got that one down. And then, I don't force her to eat it. It's just going to lead to a bad experience. I just wait and try it again later."

Getting toddlers to try things and take that first bite can be difficult. "She loves fruit. So as long as there's fruit on the plate, in a bowl, next to her, I know she'll eat that. . . . You just have to put something new next to something she recognizes. She needs that push through," says Gross. He also finds things he knows she likes and then "mixes in a few things." I tried this and found it to be true for Cody. I'd also make bites for Cody on the fork and feed them to him so he could taste ingredients together. I'd tell him that meat with sauce on it tastes really good, or that asparagus with melted Parmesan cheese on top is yummy together. Studies also show that children begin to associate foods with experiences. Children who are fed a new food followed by something sweet, like peaches, are more likely to accept the new food—they will build an association between the new food and the pleasant experience with the sweet peaches.

There are many other strategies for dealing with a picky eater. Most important is remembering not to struggle over food. If you find yourself getting frustrated, it's best to retreat for the moment. Children of all ages respond badly to what they perceive as bullying and shaming. A child may decide she doesn't like a food because she associates it with an unpleasant experience. Try to stay good-humored and lighthearted when you talk with your children about food.

Avoiding Food Wars

As adults we eat conscientiously, thinking about health, but kids are notoriously picky eaters and simply won't eat things that don't appeal to them. They are too young for reasoning, and it is not a strategy that works well. Also, kids at this age quickly learn the power of refusing a food, and the classic "picky eater" struggle can ensue because they begin to assert their independence. "They need to be able to control their world," says Cynthia Epps, an infant-feeding specialist. I've always relied on making things fun with Cody and using games and distraction, knowing that bribing and begging would be counterproductive, unpleasant, and uncomfortable for both of us. Many of our meals start off with "no" but end with an empty plate.

Sortun gets creative by playing upon her daughter's imagination. This is a very imaginative age, and one day her daughter called a cucumber stick "yucky" even though it has been a repeated staple that they grow on their farm and that she loves. Instead of taking the challenge head-on, Sortun playfully said, "It's not a cucumber, it's a bridge." Seeing the cucumber as something fun motivated Siena to pick it up and start eating it.

Nguyen creates a feeling of trust with her son, James: "I say 'try it once, if you don't like it, spit it out,' and I hold my hand out for him to spit it into. With every new dish, I say, 'James, here's a little piece, try it. Here's my hand, if you don't like it, spit it out.' Every once in a while he says, 'OOOH, I like it.'"

"They are very strong-willed little people," says Gross. "I decided that my daughter and I have a better relationship because I don't talk to her like she's two. I talk to her like she's twenty-two, and it seems to work out really well for me. I don't get nearly as upset about things. I just tell her like it is," he says.

"Food is the very first opportunity toddlers have to control what they do. It's not that they don't like the food you put out in front of them; they just rather

you don't put food on a plate right in front of them. Instead, put an empty plate in front of them and a serving plate with food just beyond and let them pick and choose family style," explains Epps. Toddlers are learning that they are separate beings and can affect their world, and so they embrace and test this power constantly. It's best to give toddlers control of the space right in front of them—what's in arm's reach when they sit at the table. It doesn't work to simply put a plate in front of them and expect them to comply. Epps suggests that a more clever way to acknowledge this new power they have to exert control is to instead play on their curious nature by putting things within their reach and allowing them to take for themselves.

"Knowing how to get around food wars is key. . . . It's knowing how to keep them on track, how to stay cool, how not to fight with them," says Epps. She teaches that a parent has the responsibility for what, where, and when the child eats, but the child is responsible for whether or not he is going to eat and how much he eats. "As parents, it's real hard to back off and allow that to happen," continues Epps. "What you need to know is how you get into a rhythm of breakfast, snack, lunch, snack, dinner through the day so that if any one of those breaks down, there's a snack or a meal coming within a couple of hours." She defines a snack as the leftovers of the previous meal or a substantial food instead of the easy to grab but nutritionally incomplete prepackaged foods like cheese puffs or dried cereal.

"Sometimes, I get a little frustrated with Madi when she hasn't eaten all day, and I find myself falling into that trap of trying to get her to eat more than she

ALEJANDRO ALCOCER was born in Mexico and has worked in renowned restaurants all over the world. He infuses the food at Green Brown Orange, his tiny, upscale neighborhood cafe, catering company, and marketplace on Manhattan's Lower East Side, with an eclectic mix of earthy, local flavors and worldly nuance. Alcocer loves to travel around the world with his children. He is a single father of two boys: Joaquin Cristobel in New York and Constantin in Berlin. Alcocer says of being around restaurants, "It's a lifestyle. We grow our own produce. The restaurant is an offshoot of a catering business and a place to showcase what we do."

wants. But if she eats only two bites at dinner, she eats only two bites. Then, at breakfast, I'll make her some eggs and give her a banana, and she'll go to town on it—I think that's what you need to do. Parents get frustrated that kids won't eat what they want them to at dinnertime, and they think, gosh, they can't go to bed without eating," says Colby Garrelts. Sortun says of her daughter, "She is not a big eater—she snacks

a lot . . . she's a grazer, she doesn't eat a lot at once." Even if kids don't eat a lot, it's important for children at this age to learn to sit at the table, because "eating around the house and roaming, they become grazers. We want to make sure we are not starting a bad habit early on," says Kravich.

Getting Kids to the Table and Trying Foods

Some fussy eating is rooted in behavior—children at this age prefer to play rather than sit and eat, and they have a hard time stopping a fun game. Many toddlers have trouble making transitions between activities, and going from playtime to mealtime is no exception. To help Cody get to the table to eat, I encouraged him to bring things that he was playing with, like his toy dinosaur, to the table with him—"because he's hungry, too," I would say playfully. I would ask his dinosaur, "Are you hungry, dinosaur?" Sometimes, to get Cody focused on eating, I'd ask his belly if it was hungry. "Knock, knock, Cody's belly, are you hungry?" I'd then exclaim, "Your belly's hungry, he just told me, he wants some soup."

To get kids to eat, chefs also talk about how important it is to convey the sensory appeal of foods to kids. McNamara says, "There's a way of holding food, showing it, and enjoying watching your kids look at it and try it," she says. Otsuka adds, "I talk about colors with my daughter. She understands what she likes by colors. Green needs to be on the plate." And if his daughter doesn't like something, he says, "I'll just step away from it for a few days, and then maybe bring it back and try again later." For Cody, I expanded the basic

> "It's tough with the little ones because most of the not eating stuff is psychological until they get to that age where they feel more comfortable trying things."
>
> —Andrea Curto-Randazzo, Miami chef

repertoire of food bite sounds to include racecars and rocket ships.

Sometimes peer pressure helps. If your child observes that an unusual or exotic food is desirable to others, he'll be more likely to try it. Alcocer relates a story about visiting Mozambique with Constantin, where everyone ate a certain fatty and smelly fish. "It was a completely different fish experience than Constantin was used to. But he saw that the local children and their parents were enjoying it—so he began to enjoy it, too."

We have to balance our kids' training between two main points they must learn: to listen to their own bodies to know when they are hungry or full, and to eat regularly according to the schedule of meals that we eat as a society—breakfast, lunch, and dinner. "I don't want to tell James to eat when he is not hungry," says Nguyen.

"When Madi is hungry, she eats," says Megan Garrelts.

"It's not always going to be at the same time that we are all hungry, but she eats the stuff I want her to eat when she is hungry," adds Colby Garrelts.

"Some days, like yesterday, she came home from preschool and wanted cereal for lunch and

MARC MURPHY's cuisine is thoughtful but casual and includes rustic Italian dishes and French bistro fare at his three New York–area neighborhood restaurants: Landmarc Tribeca, Landmarc Time Warner, and Ditch Plains. Murphy is one of the frequent judges on the Food Network show *Chopped* and has competed on *Iron Chef*. Murphy has two daughters, Callen and Campbell. He says proudly of Callen, "One of her favorite things to eat when she was four was fennel salad with smoked oysters." They go to the market together and see what's good, and that's what they cook at home.

that's what she wanted," says Megan. "You know we go through that as adults, too. Some nights I come home and I want oatmeal for dinner or something out of the ordinary. I remember sometimes my mom would make us breakfast for dinner, like pancakes and eggs, just because that was the fun. Even though they are just little people and they don't communicate very well, kids still have cravings and wants just like we do as adults."

•• **Share your food.** Toddlers mimic and model their behavior on you. They are naturally interested in the foods you're eating. "It's like learning how to talk: They talk like we talk. They eat what we eat," says Chef Marc Murphy.

•• **Toddlers like to be helpful and involved.** Let your child help shop for and prepare a meal, and talk about the fruits and vegetables as you go: what's fresh, what looks good, how you will combine them. Let him help you pick the apples from the bin in the market. Ask him what he wants to eat, both at the market and at home. At home, give him a safe and kid-friendly task like washing the vegetables. When he becomes more coordinated, let him mix, measure, pour, and grate.

•• **Kids learn by doing.** Murphy has a special children's stepstool, designed for the kitchen, called a "learning tower." It allows his daughter to climb up and be at a safe height to stand at the stove. They make omelettes together.

•• **Make food fun.** Chef Joan McNamara says food should be all about "fun and love." Boys are often interested in cars, trains, and airplanes, so use the age-old game of "here comes the train." Do train bites with train sounds, car bites with car sounds, and plane bites with plane sounds. Chef Alejandro Alcocer plays an octopus-eating-shark game at the table with his son. I like to bring a toy dinosaur to the table and have the dinosaur ask Cody to take a bite.

•• **Be open and experimental.** Try new things. Chef Eric Bromberg says, "We make our own pancakes and let them put in any ingredients they want. Sometimes the pancakes are green and disgusting, sometimes they're black and stick to the pan, and sometimes they're light and fluffy. It's all part of experimenting: seeing what you like and how you make stuff. It adds a whole new level of interest—that food is a cool thing. It's entertaining!"

•• **Play smelling games.** Chef Michael Otsuka takes his daughter, Olivia, into their garden to smell and identify herbs. They incorporate those herbs into their meals. Experiments suggest that the sense of smell accounts for up to 90 percent of our perception of flavor and lots of flavors, like vanilla and tarragon, are purely smell. While taste preferences are inborn, according to Marcia Pelchat, a biopsychologist, aromas seem to be learned and preferences are a matter of culture and experience. It's fun and surprising to shake and sniff, or scratch and sniff, foods like cinnamon sticks, fennel seeds, and cumin. Warming foods releases their aromas. Take, for example, the difference between raw garlic and garlic that is sautéed.

- **Hold off on ready-made meals, fast foods, and sugars.** Let your child's palate develop from the flavor and nutrition of the food you make for him. It establishes a foundation for her understanding of what constitutes "good" food. The processed chemical flavors of candy, soda, and junk food easily overwhelm the simple flavors of real foods like corn and broccoli.

- **Talk about it.** Chefs constantly discuss ingredients, menus, and recipes with their children. This kind of exposure is a form of education. McNamara enthuses, "We love talking about food!"

- **Eat at ethnic restaurants.** "Dining in those restaurants is a different experience from dining in a fine-dining restaurant where the formality of the meal is a little more precise," says Chef Cathal Armstrong. "There's a variety of unique flavors with each cuisine and it can be good exposure." Also, kids will often try new and more adventurous things when dining out because it's part of the experience. "I don't know if it's because that place has such different things, she feels comfortable trying it, but she'll go, 'Yeah, I'll try that.' She's always a little more adventurous when we go to that specific restaurant," says Chef Andrea Curto-Randazzo.

- **Distract them.** Not talking about the problem at hand can be a useful tool. Occasionally Cody will say his food is "yucky" when we sit down to dinner, and then he'll say, "I don't like it." I just eat my dinner and talk about something else. He'll stall and wait to see if he gets a reaction, and then slowly on his own he'll start to eat. I can also break into singing his favorite song and he'll smile and forget all about yucky. Another game I play is "open your mouth and close your eyes and I will give you a big surprise." We'll try to guess what food from his plate was on the bite. I tell him, "You have to chew and swallow to figure it out."

- **Introduce the food to them.** When there's soup that Cody's hesitant to eat, I give him toast to go with it and I make a big silly surprise face and dip the toast in the soup. He'll eat the toast, then jump in to eat some of the soup. I'll also start counting the carrot pieces floating in the soup, and we'll play a numbers game of swirling them and getting them on the spoon.

- **Use quality ingredients.** The better your ingredients, the simpler and less time-consuming your food preparation can be and the more flavorful your food will be. Produce that is old loses its flavor and tastes starchy and wooden.

- **Try to avoid being a short-order cook.** Feed your kids what you eat, or make simplified versions of adult foods. It's easier and more efficient than cooking to order, and it creates a nice sense of family and togetherness.

Healthy Eating

What we eat plays a big role in how we feel. Sugars, including those found in fruit juice, have a profound effect on our bodies, affecting brain concentration and energy levels. Chefs know that a child who is ingesting sugary snacks and drinks is going to behave differently. "Joaquin is starting to go through the terrible twos," says New York chef Alcocer. "We're careful about what he eats. We keep him away from sugar. We give him a nonsugary cereal in the morning. At night we give him starch and vegetables so it's easier for him to transition into sleep."

Most chefs don't consume fast food on a regular basis, and they pass their attitudes down to their children. "My kids don't like McDonald's," says Forley. "It probably rubbed off from us; I'm sure we've said bad things about McDonald's in front of them." Forley doesn't keep packaged or precooked food in their house, knowing that ready-made foods taste different than foods we cook ourselves and are usually made from ingredients that are lower in quality and freshness. Prepackaged foods contain more sugar, salt, and chemicals to flavor and preserve the food. Staying away from those foods is a great way to stay healthy.

It's not just a matter of limiting sugar and fast food. Even cooking at home has changed. "I'm not allowed to use butter anymore," Murphy says ruefully. "My wife has informed me that the butter part of our relationship is over. The idea of a healthy breakfast has changed. When we were kids, it was eggs, toast with butter, orange juice, and bacon. We've learned so much more about what's bad for us. The first couple

of years are when kids build up their fat cells. So we really limit the fatty or fat-producing foods. We have to be careful."

While I know using a stick of butter in a pan to cook mushrooms is way too much fat to be healthy, I still serve Cody butter on his toast and even put a small amount in our home-cooked dishes and even on vegetables from time to time. Kravich says, "I use some butter on vegetables like butternut squash for kids so that it feels creamy and it tastes yummy. As far as dessert goes, we'll make things like an apple crisp; I just don't put a lot of sweetening in it." Kravich also advises parents to feed their children whole grains instead of white rice and breads and pasta made from white flour. Those foods aren't good for the digestion, she says. She advises feeding kids different-colored rice like red rice and black rice or rice that has a variety of colors mixed together.

Berley made lots of quick pickles with vegetables like string beans and cauliflower for his children. Pickled foods are not cooked but are preserved in vinegar and contain the same nutrition as raw vegetables. Kids love pickles, they are crunchy and salty and you can make quick refrigerator pickles at home in different flavors by adding different herbs and spices, or you can keep them plain if that's what your kids prefer.

Processed foods usually include flavoring agents that make them taste differently from home-cooked foods. Becoming too accustomed to these unnatural flavors can make it harder to appreciate the flavors of wholesome foods. Keep use of processed foods to a minimum and teach your kids to be flexible eaters with discerning palates. "I'd rather give my

PETER BERLEY is the former executive chef of the renowned vegan restaurant Angelica Kitchen in New York City. He is not a vegetarian himself but is known for his savvy about vegetarian cooking and won a James Beard award for his book *The Modern Vegetarian Kitchen*. He has two other popular cookbooks and also works as a culinary educator. He is knowledgeable about macrobiotic eating and raised his family on its principles. He has two adult daughters, Kayla and Emma. Berley says, "I study about food, I've never been into studying nutrition. I've been very skeptical about the science of nutrition only because a lot of it is so much based on one book that analyzes nutritional components in food—there's only one book that everything is based on—all the how much vitamin C is in something, how much vitamin A is in something—that all comes from only one source, which is really not very accurate. That's part of it. The other thing is, I found that to think that way is very analytical and very cerebral, and I've always felt that it's best to see how you feel with what you eat."

Chef Peter Berley and daughter Kayla : Cam Camaren

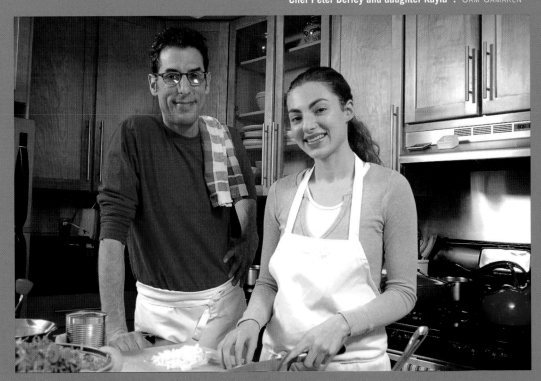

son a bar of good chocolate than something that is rainbow-colored and has high-fructose corn syrup in it," says Nguyen.

Megan Garrelts is the pastry chef at her and her husband's restaurant. How does she moderate the amount of sweets Madi eats? "I try to not have too many conversations. I just tell her no and we move on. I'll change the topic," says Megan.

Eating at Restaurants

"I think it's important to expose your kids to restaurants," says Megan Garrelts. "When Madi was an infant even, we brought her in all the time—she would sleep in her car seat. I don't think it's appropriate to take infants out to twelve-course tasting menus every night, but, at the same time, if you shelter them from ever being in normal day-to-day restaurants and socializing with people on that level, you're adding fuel to the fire."

Children learn table manners and etiquette at restaurants. "Madi's very good at restaurants," continues Megan. "She always wants a napkin because she sees everyone around her with a napkin. It's funny because we didn't teach her that. When we eat in the lounge at the restaurant, the server will bring her a napkin and silverware, and she has to have that stuff before we eat. She understands everything that goes into having a meal, sitting down and waiting for her food."

"When we go out to a restaurant, we're there to eat," says Chef Andrea Curto-Randazzo. "I remember when I was growing up, you went out to eat, you sat in your seat, you weren't climbing everywhere or you got *the look*. I think, also, when I was little I had an appreciation for food—I remember telling my dad, 'I want the big person's size.' It would always be, 'Baby, you can have whatever you want.' I was excited about that. I try to make my children feel the same way. They are super excited to go out to dinner; they know it's a treat and it's special, so we are there to eat. The baby is into the sugar packets, but she's two and a half, so you gotta give in to a little something."

Eating at restaurants is a good time to try new foods. Pelchat paints a picture of how parents she has known may have conditioned their children to become picky. She says, "While they were willing to eat at a Brazilian restaurant, they didn't order the *feijoada,* the scary dish. They ordered steaks or something. Both of them sent their food back several times with minor complaints. Plus, they didn't eat with their kids. That kind of made sense to me that their son would end up being picky."

Try to make eating out an opportunity for your family to try new things. Make a point of ordering something adventurous—even if it's only a side dish or an unusual appetizer. Try ordering a number of smaller plates that you can all taste and share.

chicken and rice with vegetable gravy

{ ZACK GROSS }

SERVES 4

I love chicken and gravy. This gravy is easy to make and so delicious. Lots of gravies are made with flour, but this gravy with cream has a satisfying rich and delicate flavor. Chef Zack Gross suggests serving with jasmine rice.

4 chicken breasts, bone in and skin on
Salt and pepper
1 tablespoon olive oil
1 onion, peeled and chopped
2 carrots, peeled and chopped
2 stalks celery, chopped
¾ cup chopped mushrooms
2 cups chicken stock
2 tablespoons fresh thyme
2 tablespoons fresh rosemary
¼ cup heavy cream (or crème fraîche or a pat of
    butter—but not milk)

1. Preheat oven to 325°F.

2. Season the chicken with salt and pepper. Heat a large straight-sided, ovenproof skillet over medium-high heat, and when the pan is hot, add the oil. Brown the chicken skin-side down in batches if necessary so as not to crowd the pan, about 5 minutes each side. Remove browned pieces to a plate as you brown the next batch.

3. When all the chicken is browned, turn the breasts skin-side up and snuggle them all together in the pan. Add the chopped vegetables to the pan in and around the chicken, and put the pan in the oven, uncovered, for about 15 minutes.

4. Remove the pan from the oven to the stovetop and remove the chicken to a plate. Spoon out or pour off all but a tablespoon or so of fat, leaving the vegetables in the pan.

5. Put the pan back on the stovetop, over low heat, and pour the chicken stock into the pan, stirring and scraping to incorporate any browned bits off the bottom of the pan. Add the fresh herbs and cream (if using butter, mix in at the end, off heat) to stock. Raise the heat and reduce the liquid by about half, until thickened, about 8 to 10 minutes.

6. When thickened, pour the gravy into a food processor or blender and pulse until smooth. If using a blender, leave some room at the top and pulse the blender without the very top piece on to let the steam escape. Finally, season with salt and pepper and pour the gravy over the chicken and serve.

Note: You can easily make this with skinless, boneless chicken breasts also.

chicken cassoulet with white beans and bacon

{ COLBY GARRELTS }

SERVES 4

A cassoulet is a deeply flavorful and satisfying meal. Usually it is cooked and then allowed to rest overnight to deepen the flavors before reheating and serving. I find myself making this dish on a Sunday afternoon when we feel like being homebodies, playing board games or reading lots of books. Any leftovers are delicious the next day for lunch with a salad or mixed into some broth. Done right, the flavors meld together and the beans are soft and creamy. Cody likes the tomato-y beans, and sometimes we serve this with wheat toast and call it "beans on toast." If you have sausages on hand instead of bacon, go ahead and use them or any other meat you have around.

4 slices French bread or other similar bread, cut into small cubes

3 bacon slices, coarsely chopped into ¼- to ½-inch pieces

1½ pounds chicken breasts or thighs, cut into ¾-inch-thick cubes (pound breast to an even thickness before cubing)

1 tablespoon olive oil

1 medium shallot, chopped

3 garlic cloves, chopped

2 teaspoons chopped fresh oregano

2 teaspoons chopped fresh thyme

¼ teaspoon dried crushed red pepper (optional)

1 cup chicken stock

1 15-ounce can great northern beans, drained

1 14½-ounce can diced tomatoes in juice

3 tablespoons tomato paste

½ teaspoon ground allspice

Salt and pepper

2 tablespoons olive oil

½ cup freshly grated Parmesan cheese

2 tablespoons chopped fresh parsley

1. Preheat oven to 200°F. Spread the bread cubes out onto a baking sheet and bake until dry and crumbly, about 10 minutes, stirring halfway through. Remove from oven and when cool, crush in your hands to make coarse crumbs.

2. Cook bacon in a medium-size, heavy ovenproof Dutch oven (or straight-sided skillet with a tight-fitting lid) over medium-high heat until brown and crisp, about 4 minutes. Using a slotted spoon, transfer bacon to a bowl.

3. Add chicken to pot to brown, but do not cook through. Using a slotted spoon, transfer the chicken to the bowl with the bacon. Pour off the fat from the pot.

4. Turn heat down to low and add the olive oil, shallot, and garlic to pot and sauté until beginning to soften, about 10 minutes. Stir in oregano, thyme, and red pepper. Add chicken stock and beans and then turn up the heat until liquid is reduced below beans and is thickened, about 15 minutes.

5. Turn oven up to 350°F.

6. Stir in tomatoes with juices, tomato paste, and allspice. Return chicken and bacon to pot. Season cassoulet with salt and pepper. Taste to test for flavor and add more salt and pepper if needed. Bring to boil.

7. Cover pot and transfer to preheated oven; bake 30 minutes. Remove pot from the oven.

8. If making to serve at a later time, uncover pot and cool the cassoulet 1 hour at room temperature. Then refrigerate, uncovered, until cold. Once cold, cover and keep refrigerated. When ready to use, rewarm, covered, in 375°F oven about 40 minutes, adding more broth if necessary.

9. Increase oven temperature to 400°F. In a bowl, mix bread crumbs with Parmesan cheese and season with salt and pepper. Sprinkle over warm cassoulet. Bake until bread crumb topping is golden brown, about 10 minutes covered and another 5 to 10 minutes uncovered. Sprinkle cassoulet with parsley and serve.

Note: If you have leftover chicken that is already cooked, you can use that in the recipe instead of raw chicken. Cut the chicken into cubes and skip the step of browning; add cooked chicken cubes to the bowl with the cooked bacon.

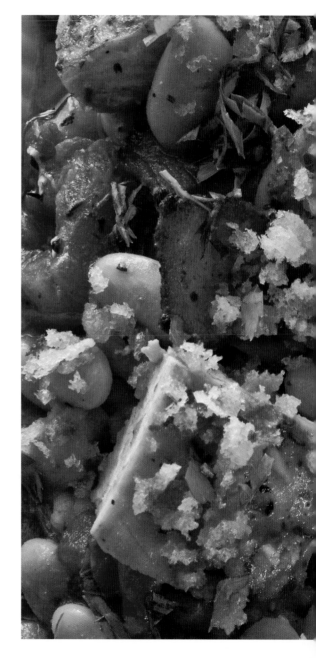

hot dogs with homemade relish and carrot sticks

{ ZACK GROSS }

SERVES 4

Hot dogs are a swift, unfussy, hit-the-spot lunch or dinner. Chef Zack Gross says he likes Hebrew National hot dogs and potato rolls. He boils his dogs, and then keeps them warm in the water while he makes the relish. It's worth the extra time to cut the onions and pickles very fine, especially for kids. I can't stop looking for a snack to have with this relish when I make it, and when my friend Piper comes over, we cut the hot dogs lengthwise and then into small folded bites that we eat like pretty canapés with a dollop of relish in the middle.

¼ cup finely chopped red onion
¼ cup finely chopped yellow onion
1 tablespoon red wine vinegar
1 tablespoon brown sugar
2 tablespoons water
¼ cup finely chopped dill pickles
1½ teaspoons mustard or more to your liking (yellow, Dijon, or brown)
4 best-quality buns
4 best-quality hot dogs, cooked
Bunch of carrots, peeled and cut into sticks, for serving

1. To make the relish, heat a small sauté pan over medium heat and cook the onions with the vinegar, brown sugar, and water until the onions are soft and most of the water is absorbed, about 10 minutes. Remove from heat to a bowl and combine with the pickles and mustard.

2. To steam the buns, put the heated hot dogs in the buns and put them back into the bun bag and tie closed; let stand about 2 minutes. Remove to a plate and serve carrot sticks on the side.

steamed black cod with ginger broth, lime, and noodles

{ COLBY GARRELTS }

This is Chef Colby Garrelts's favorite meal in the world. Mine, too. The broth is fantastic and even better if you make the stock yourself, which is as easy as throwing some fish bones (or shrimp shells) in a pot with water and an onion and some of the other ingredients from the list below for 20 minutes. Don't boil the water, or the stock will get cloudy. We bring both the soy sauce and the sesame oil to the table, so Cody can pour a bit extra into the soup himself. The same recipe can also be made with chicken stock and boneless chicken breast, but omit the fish sauce.

I also like Colby's clever method of using a pie dish to steam the fish in the pot with the broth.

6 ounces rice noodles

1½ cups snow peas, ends trimmed

1 cup shredded carrots

4 cups good quality fresh fish stock (clam juice or even chicken stock can be substituted)

1 tablespoon grated peeled fresh ginger

1 tablespoon toasted sesame oil

1 tablespoon soy sauce

1 teaspoon fish sauce, Three Crabs brand recommended (optional)

5 tablespoons fresh cilantro, divided

4 5-ounce black cod or halibut fillets

Salt and pepper

2 tablespoons chopped green onion

2 tablespoons fresh lime juice

1 tablespoon chopped fresh mint

1. Gather a large pot with a lid to make the soup, a steamer that can fit inside the pot, and a 9-inch pie dish to place the fish in.

2. In a second pot, boil the noodles in salted water for 3 minutes. Place snow peas and carrots in a colander, drain noodles over them, and rinse and divide among 4 bowls.

3. In the large pot, place the fish stock, ginger, sesame oil, soy sauce, fish sauce, and 3 tablespoons cilantro; bring broth to a boil.

4. Add steamer rack or basket to pot. Place the fish in the glass pie dish, sprinkle with salt and pepper, and place pie dish on top of steamer rack. Cover pot and steam fish just until opaque in center, about 6 minutes for cod and 8 minutes for halibut. Serve with sauce and noodles; garnish with 2 tablespoons cilantro, green onions, lime juice, and mint.

Note: It's worth getting Thai rice noodles. Rice pasta cooks in a different way.

red bean and walnut spread

{ ANA SORTUN }

SERVES 8

At her restaurant, Oleanna, in Cambridge Massachusetts, Chef Ana Sortun serves this popular dip with homemade string cheese and bread. To prepare it, Sortun spreads the dip out on plastic wrap, tops with herbs, pomegranate molasses, and pomegranate seeds, and rolls the whole thing up. She then serves it in slices. We make the dip plain, spread it on Wasa Lite crackers, and use the herbs and pomegranate seeds on top. Cody didn't like it right away, but the next day he asked for it, talked about how much he liked it, and wanted more.

1 cup dark red kidney beans, soaked overnight and
    rinsed well

3 cups water

¼ white onion, minced

1 bay leaf

¾ cup walnuts

4 tablespoons butter

½ teaspoon chopped garlic

Salt and pepper to taste

2 teaspoons chopped dill

2 teaspoons chopped mint or basil

2 teaspoons chopped flat-leaf parsley

2 teaspoons pomegranate molasses (you can find this
    at Whole Foods or similar markets)

Bread, crackers, and string cheese for serving

Garnish for older children and adults: toasted walnuts
    and pomegranate seeds

1. Combine beans, water, onions, and bay leaf in a saucepan and bring to a boil. Turn heat down to low and simmer until tender, about an hour.

2. Heat oven to 350°F. Spread the walnuts out on a baking tray and toast for about 8 to 10 minutes, stirring once, and checking frequently until toasted.

3. Drain beans well and discard bay leaf. In a food processor fitted with a metal blade, puree the beans with walnuts, butter, chopped garlic, salt, and pepper until smooth and creamy.

4. Mix chopped herbs together and put aside a small amount for garnish. Blend the rest into the beans and add a splash of water if the mixture is too thick.

5. Season with salt and pepper and serve on warmed bread slices or crackers. Drizzle with pomegranate molasses and sprinkle with herb mix.

6. Serve next to some string cheese. For older children and adults, top with walnuts and pomegranate seeds.

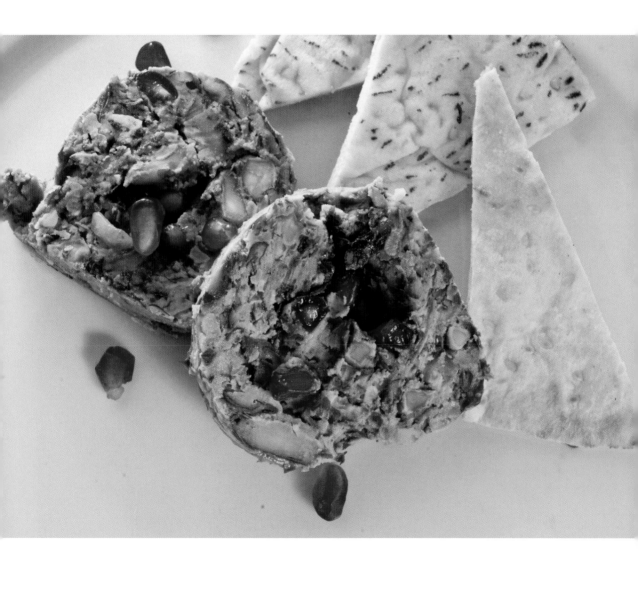

ratatouille with balsamic vinegar, honey, and basil

{ DIANE FORLEY }

SERVES 4–6

This dish is just delicious—the balsamic, honey, and basil are unique additions.

1 onion, diced

1 eggplant, diced,

1 red pepper, diced

2 zucchini, diced

¼ cup olive oil

1 tablespoon ground fennel seed

1 tablespoon ground coriander seed

1 tablespoon salt

1 cup tomato sauce

2 tablespoons balsamic vinegar

2 tablespoons honey

1 bunch basil leaves (15 leaves), chopped

1. Preheat oven to 375°F.

2. Toss vegetables with olive oil, spices, and salt; place on foil-lined baking sheet and bake until vegetables are browned, about 45 minutes to 1 hour, stirring often to cook evenly.

3. Remove vegetables from oven and transfer to medium-size pot. Add tomato sauce, vinegar, and honey and let cook over low heat until mixture softens, about 10 minutes.

4. Remove from heat and add chopped basil and serve.

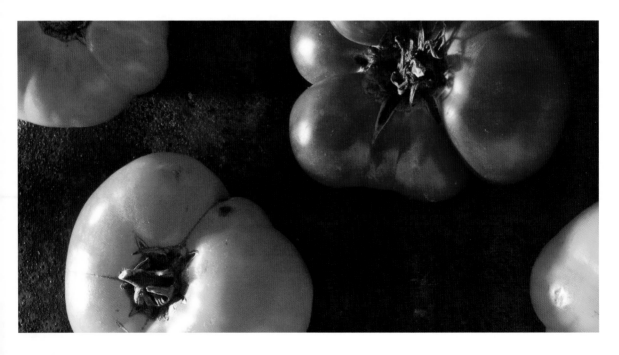

nori chips

{ PETER BERLEY }

SERVES 4

Chef Peter Berley's children grew up on these tasty nori seaweed chips the way most kids grow up eating potato chips. Nori are thin sheets of dried seaweed commonly used for wrapping sushi. Nori has lots of protein, and few other foods contain as many vitamins and minerals. They can be found in the Asian section of the grocery store. Nori chips are super fast and easy to make. I like them with sesame oil brushed on after baking. You can store them for several days, but when we make them, we never have any left!

5 nori sheets (one package)
1 teaspoon olive oil
Salt for sprinkling
Sesame oil (optional)

1. Preheat oven to 300°F.

2. Lay the nori sheets out on a baking tray—you can cut some in half to fit your baking tray. Brush them lightly with olive oil and sprinkle lightly with salt.

3. Bake for 15 to 20 minutes, until crisp like a potato chip. Brush lightly with sesame oil if you like. Break into bite-size pieces and serve.

Tip: You can make incredibly crunchy and delicate kale chips the same way, at the same time, but keep a close eye on them so they don't burn.

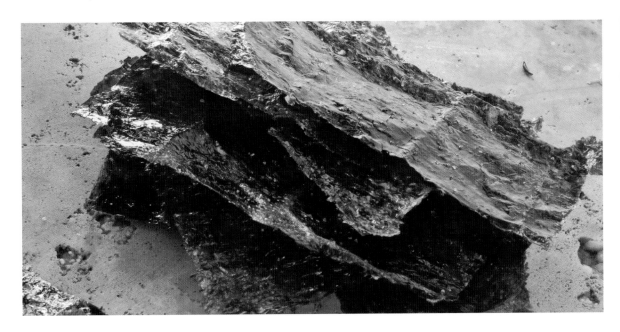

macaroni and cheese

{ JOAN MCNAMARA }

SERVES 10

"My grandson eats our macaroni and cheese, that we have here, that was my mother's recipe. . . . I would make that for my kids," says Joan McNamara, founder of Joan's on Third cafe in Los Angeles. She says she learned to cook from her mother, who would encourage her cooking and tell her just not to be afraid, **"just go ahead and try."** Her macaroni and cheese is unlike any other. She explains: **"Most people do a roux (a cooked mixture of flour and butter) in macaroni and cheese—and this one doesn't. It's just everything thrown in the pot—you boil the noodles, then put in milk and butter and any kind of cheese you want, put it in the oven, and it's done. My mother would say, 'just add the milk'— it would be swimming in milk. *Swimming!* It looked like you had put all that macaroni in this pool of milk, and she'd say, 'Don't be afraid to put in too much, it will absorb into the thing,' and sure enough it did."**

1½ tablespoons salt

1 pound pasta (elbow macaroni, fusilli, or any shape desired)

2 ounces (4 tablespoons) butter

3¾ cups whole milk

6 ounces ricotta or small curd cottage cheese

3 ounces cream cheese

12 ounces Monterey Jack cheese, shredded

20 ounces Old Amsterdam Gouda (see note at right), shredded, divided

Salt and pepper to taste

1. Preheat oven to 350°F.

2. Bring a large pot of water to a boil. Add 1½ tablespoons salt, and when the water returns to a boil, add the pasta and cook until just tender. While the pasta cooks, measure and put in a large bowl the butter, milk, ricotta or cottage cheese, cream cheese, Monterey Jack cheese, and 12 ounces of Old Amsterdam Gouda (reserve the rest for the topping). When the pasta is tender, drain well and add warm to the other ingredients. Season with salt and pepper. Gently mix everything together, leaving some chunks of cheese visible.

3. Pour the mixture into 9 x 11-inch baking pan. Top with the remaining Gouda. You can store this in the refrigerator until you are ready to cook. Bake for 30 to 40 minutes, or until beautifully golden.

4. Serve hot or at room temperature.

Note: Aged Gouda cheeses have a more intense butterscotch-caramel flavor than regular Gouda cheeses. Old Amsterdam is an award-winning brand of Gouda cheese, aged 18 months and known for its rich flavor. It is rich, but not dry or salty like other matured cheeses. It can be found at fine cheese shops as well as places liked Trader Joe's. If you can't find Old Amsterdam, you can substitute with half the quantity of another high-quality aged Gouda.

Tip: Try making this in muffin wrappers in a muffin pan for smaller portions and easy serving at a party.

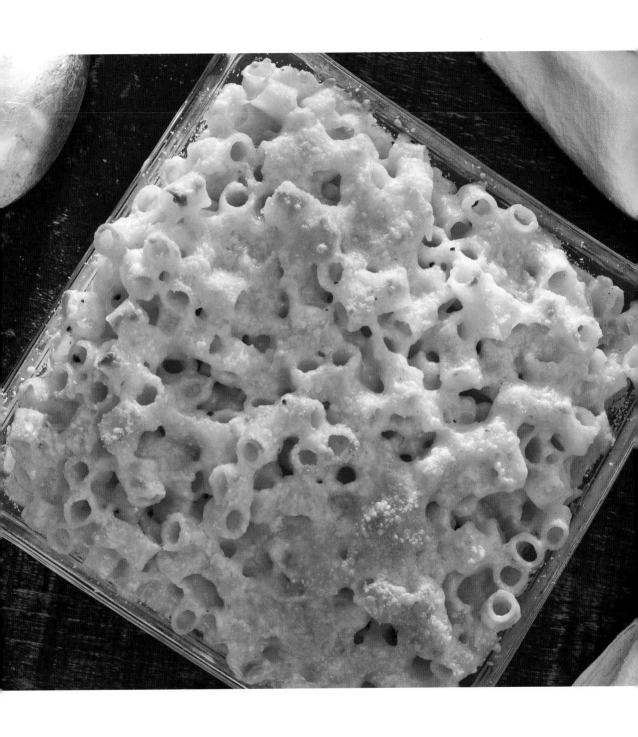

whole grain sesame scallion pancakes with tofu

{ DIANE FORLEY }

I sometimes make these as part of Cody's packed lunch, and sometimes we make them together and shape them like dinosaurs with a cookie cutter. Cody doesn't always like the texture of the soft tofu in the pancakes, even if I chop the tofu small, so we occasionally add chicken or fresh soybeans, called edamame. These can be made with leftover plain grains or leftover rice from a flavored rice dish—omit the soy sauce or make the grains fresh.

2 eggs

2 cups cooked grains: rice, barley, or quinoa

2 tablespoons soy sauce (if using plain grains)

1 tablespoon sesame oil

1 tablespoon sliced scallions, white and light green part only (optional)

½ cup flour

Salt and pepper to taste

1 cup cubed tofu

3 tablespoons olive oil

1. In a bowl, beat eggs with a fork.

2. Add grains, soy sauce if using, sesame oil, scallions if using, flour, salt, and pepper. Gently mix in tofu.

3. Heat olive oil in an 8-inch nonstick skillet over medium heat. Scoop small portions, flatten into pancakes, and place in the pan. Cook until brown on one side, about 5 minutes. Flip carefully with a spatula and finish browning over low heat until cooked through. The pancakes can also be baked in oiled muffin tins in a 375°F oven for 20 minutes.

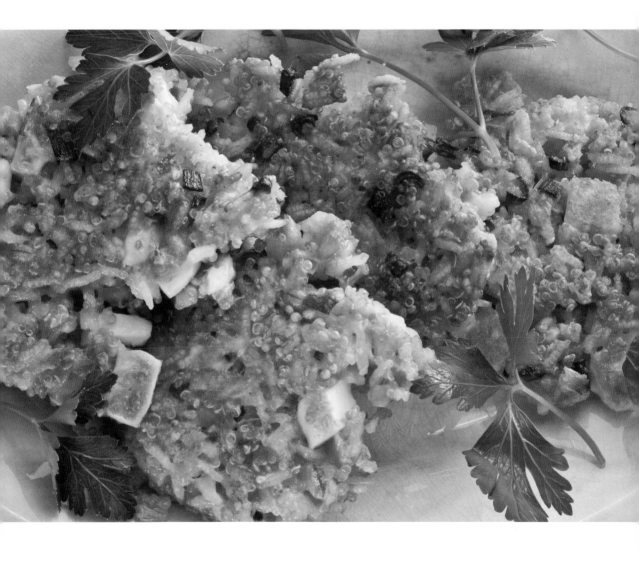

cauliflower and parmesan macaroni

{ JIMMY SCHMIDT }

SERVES 4

This is so creamy and decadent—it's a wonderful treat. You can make it in muffin tins to serve in small portions or to serve easily at a party. Parmesan cheese has a strong flavor; substitute a milder cheese for children who prefer blander flavors.

1½ tablespoons salt

2 cups elbow macaroni (preferably whole wheat or high fiber)

1 large head cauliflower, core removed, brown spots, if any, scraped off, and florets separated

1 cup half-and-half (more if necessary)

2 cups finely grated Parmesan cheese

Sea salt

1. Bring a large pot of water to a boil. Add 1½ tablespoons salt, and when the water returns to a boil, add the pasta and cook until just tender. Meanwhile, place the cauliflower florets in a colander set atop the pasta water and cover to steam the cauliflower while the pasta cooks. Turn the heat down a bit to keep the water boiling but not boiling over.

2. When the cauliflower is tender, remove it from the colander and pour it into a food processor. When the pasta is tender, drain and transfer it to a bowl.

3. Preheat oven to 400°F.

4. Puree the cauliflower with the half-and-half until smooth, then blend in 1¾ cups Parmesan cheese till smooth and thick, saving ¼ cup to sprinkle on the top before baking. Adjust seasonings as necessary with sea salt.

5. Pour the cauliflower and cheese mixture into the bowl with the pasta and fold until thoroughly combined. Adjust the texture to be slightly wet as necessary with a little additional half-and-half.

6. Pour into a casserole dish and dust the top with the remaining Parmesan cheese. Cover with foil and bake in the oven for 20 minutes. Remove the foil and bake for another 5 minutes or so, until browned on top.

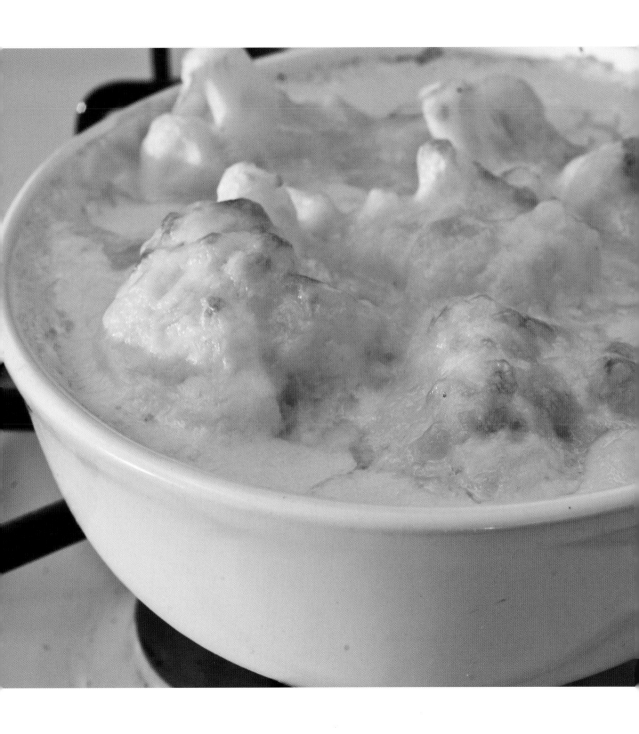

spring pea risotto with barley

{ PETER BERLEY }

SERVES 4–6

Sometimes kids need something fun to do at the table before they will settle in to eat. For this dish I gave Cody the block of Parmesan and the grater. He grated some cheese on top, mixed it in, and then started eating. This is a fast, easy meal for a babysitter to do also.

1 cup pearl barley, soaked in water to cover by 2 inches for 4 to 6 hours
½ cup finely chopped onion
1 tablespoon extra-virgin olive oil
Sea salt and freshly ground black pepper
4 cups vegetable stock
1 cup fresh peas
½ cup finely grated Parmesan cheese
1 tablespoon butter
1 teaspoon finely chopped basil or other fresh herbs (optional)

1. Drain the barley.

2. In a 2- to 3-quart saucepan, sauté the onion in olive oil with a pinch of salt over medium heat 5 to 7 minutes or until soft and translucent.

3. Stir in the barley and stock and bring to a boil. Reduce the heat and simmer for 35 minutes, stirring occasionally until most (but not all) of the liquid has been absorbed and the barley is tender.

4. Stir in the peas and cook 3 to 4 minutes or until tender. Stir in the cheese, butter, and basil. Season with salt and pepper and serve.

noodles with tahini dressing

{ ANA SORTUN }

SERVES 4

This makes a tasty and filling packed lunch. The dressing can also be used as a dip for broccoli, carrots, or cucumbers or any flat bread like pita. For a thicker dip, use less water.

1½ tablespoons salt

½ pound spaghetti (can use buckwheat noodles, rice noodles, or spaghetti)

¼ cup tahini

3 tablespoons warm water (or more for consistency)

¼ cup extra-virgin olive oil

1 teaspoon rice wine vinegar or white balsamic vinegar

2 teaspoons freshly squeezed lemon juice

½ teaspoon sugar

½ teaspoon ground cumin

1 tablespoon Greek yogurt or mayonnaise

Kosher salt to taste

Sesame seeds and finely chopped red pepper or cucumber to garnish, optional

1. Bring a large pot of water to a boil. Add 1½ tablespoons salt, and when the water returns to a boil, add the pasta and cook until just tender. When cooked, drain into a colander and rinse under cool water.

2. Meanwhile, make the tahini dressing by whisking tahini and warm water together in a bowl until smooth. Stir in the oil, vinegar, lemon juice, sugar, cumin, yogurt or mayonnaise, and salt. The dressing will last for 3 to 5 days in the refrigerator. Serve cold or at room temperature.

3. Mix the tahini dressing into cooked and rinsed pasta. Add more water if the sauce is too thick. Sprinkle the sesame seeds and chopped red pepper or cucumber on top if using and serve.

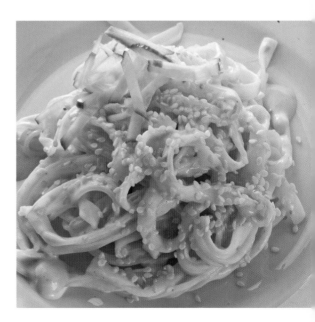

toasted mochi snack with maple syrup

{ PETER BERLEY }

{ PETER BERLEY }

SERVES 4

It's nice sometimes to have a quick sweet something without a whole lot of mess and preparation. This is both healthy and delicious. Another option for spreading on the *mochi* (and dipping!) instead of maple syrup is apple butter. Mochi is a popular Japanese food made from special sweet rice. It's made by steaming then pounding the rice into shapes and is surprisingly chewy. In Japan it is served grilled or toasted, used in soup or in desserts—soft thin sheets wrapped around ice cream are delicious. The mochi in this recipe is made with brown rice and comes in a thick sheet. When baked it puffs up so it's crispy on the outside and chewy on the inside. It can be found in a Japanese market or markets like Whole Foods or in health food stores. I like to cut the pieces up small so they are more crunchy than chewy.

1 12½-ounce package mochi
Maple syrup for drizzling and dipping

1. Preheat oven to 450°F.

2. Cut half the mochi into 1- or 2-inch squares and store the rest for future use. Spread pieces at least 1 inch apart on a baking sheet and bake 8 to 10 minutes until puffed up.

3. Drizzle on maple syrup or serve on the side for dipping.

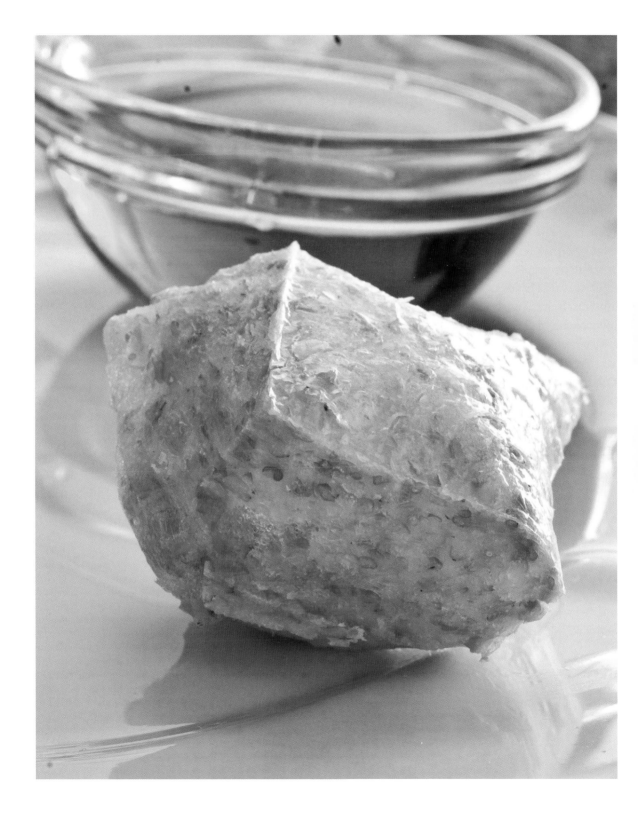

strawberry pancakes with strawberry maple syrup

{ ZACK GROSS }

SERVES 4

"Nobody has time to make pancakes from scratch with a toddler!" says Chef Zack Gross, and it's true—sometimes using a mix makes pancakes doable on a busy school day. I finally bought a double-burner skillet so I can make lots of pancakes all at once. It's fun to add strawberries or other seasonal berries, and sometimes we even add frozen cherries to ours. Gross says, "I like to put a couple of sliced strawberries into the pancake before flipping them; you can make faces and designs, whatever keeps your child's attention." He recommends Bisquick brand; I like using the different kinds of mixes from Bob's Red Mill. This sweet, buttery compote is a tasty change from maple syrup. There's no need to butter the pancakes before pouring on the sauce.

Pancake mix for at least 4 servings
4 tablespoons butter, divided
1 pint strawberries or other seasonal berries, washed and sliced, divided
2 tablespoons sugar
Juice of ½ orange, about 2 tablespoons
½ cup real maple syrup
Whipped cream (recipe below), optional

1. Follow the package instructions to make the pancake batter for at least 4 servings.

2. Ladle batter onto a hot skillet, buttered with a teaspoon or so of butter, and then gently tap the strawberry slices into the pancakes before flipping, using about ¼ of the pint.

3. In a separate pan, melt remaining butter with sugar. Add in the rest of the strawberries and the orange juice, and cook a couple of minutes.

4. Add the maple syrup and stir to combine. For special breakfasts, top with whipped cream.

Whipped Cream:
1 cup heavy cream
1 cup powdered sugar
¼ teaspoon vanilla extract

Combine all ingredients in a medium bowl and whisk until your arm hurts (or until the cream forms soft peaks).

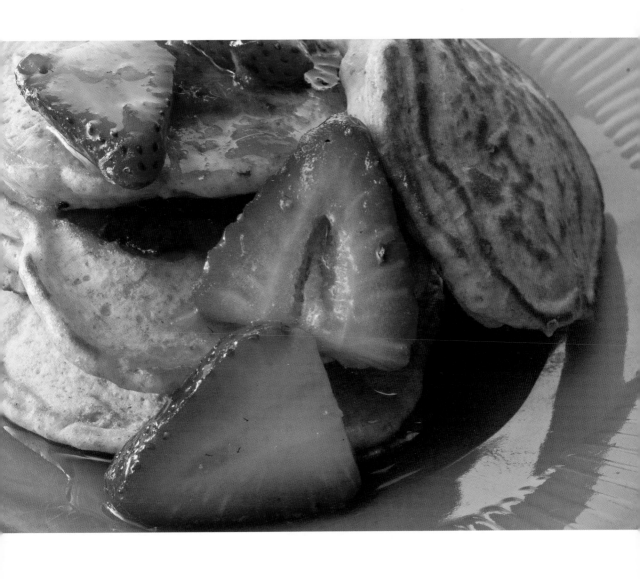

preschoolers

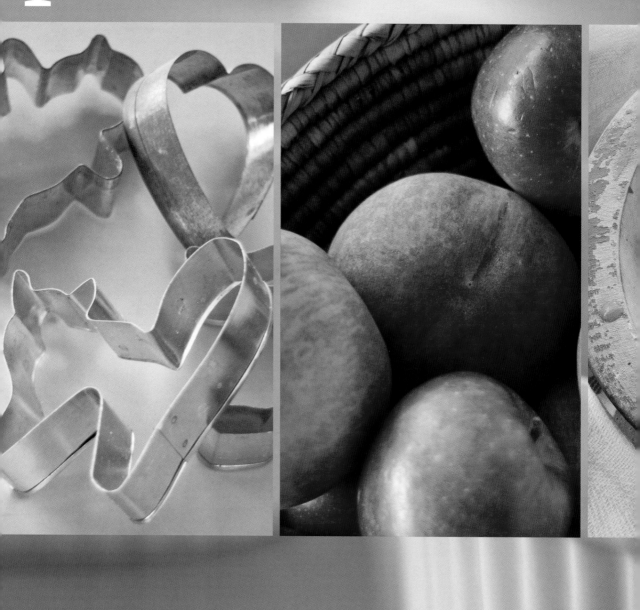

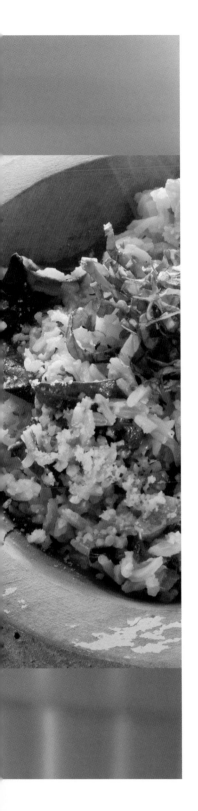

EMERGING INDEPENDENCE

ages two-and-a-half to five

All the chefs I spoke with about the preschool years agreed that this is when their kids became quirky, opinionated, and particular about the foods they ate and the way they ate them. "Children's palates change dramatically as they grow—they change as they are changing," says Chris Cosentino, executive chef at Incanto restaurant in San Francisco. "A year and a half ago, Easton loved oysters and he would down them like nobody's business. Now his palate has changed; he doesn't enjoy oysters anymore. He didn't like wasabi before; now he likes wasabi." Children at this age make decisions about eating for themselves, and it can get tricky.

Chefs' children may limit the foods they like to eat, but the foods they choose are surprising and remarkable—not at all the foods typically represented on most children's menus. Cosentino's son, Easton, loves sardines, arugula, asparagus, and sushi. Andrea Curto-Randazzo's daughter's favorite dish is rack of lamb. Siena, acclaimed Boston chef Ana Sortun's daughter, eats salads and watermelon radishes and, to Sortun's surprise, adores spicy greens. She says of her daughter, "She doesn't think any food is weird, and I love that."

It's classic that a two-year-old who eats everything will suddenly become hesitant and idiosyncratic at three years old, and about half of all children at this age do go through a tough time with food. According to Marcia Pelchat, a biopsychologist, food neophobia—when kids really don't want to eat anything new—peaks at age three and then gradually declines throughout life.

Lots of preschoolers take to eating only "white" foods like bread, pasta, potatoes, and french fries. Most, somewhere along the line, learn the word *yucky*. "It's as if children go through a tunnel at around three years old, where feeding them becomes challenging," says Floyd Cardoz, chef at New York's Tabla restaurant. "And then at five years old, they come out and are more open." It's a good time to serve more traditional and familiar foods that kids find appealing or cook meals made of simple, separate foods. Serve meals family style so kids can help themselves to the foods they are willing to eat. Miami chef Andrea Curto-Randazzo says of feeding her three daughters, "I stick to the traditional, because I'm a firm believer in those family recipes, and that stuff is simply so good. Granted, if we are having chicken chili, I might whip up my own cheddar cornbread or something." Sally Kravich, a natural health expert, advises that those starchy white foods, because they have no fiber, can be like glue in the digestion. It can make children become unhealthy. She suggests making little changes like using whole grain pasta such as those made from rice or quinoa, which are more nutritious than white-flour pasta and better for the digestive system.

How Chefs Make Food an Adventure for Their Kids

I asked chefs why their kids eat such interesting foods, and if they think there's a way that they're cooking that makes foods like vegetables palatable. The simple answer is that chefs take their children into their world of food, and, in doing so, they pass on to their children their own sense of pleasure and enthusiasm. Instead of heading to the supermarket to grab boxes and bags off of shelves, they go to the farmers' market, where kids meet farmers, taste samples, and explore inter-esting things like squash blossoms and dragon fruit. They visit local farms and orchards where children can pick food in the field—it is deeply satisfying to forage and eat a freshly picked strawberry or an apple right off a tree. They shop fresh from butchers and fishmongers, where there are curiosities like crabs—it's not just grocery shopping; it's an adventure.

Chefs teach their children, cook with them, and they cook well, using quality ingredients to make the food they cook taste better. They allow their kids to be creative with them in the kitchen, mixing their own

ingredients for making things like savory waffles with different flavors and topping combinations. Given a broad range of ingredients to choose from, children can surprise us with what they opt to eat. An example is Benchmarc executive chef Marc Murphy's daugh-ter, who visits his restaurant regularly. Murphy says, "When my daughter was three years old, she'd go into the kitchen, look at the *mise en place*, and pick up whatever she'd want, as if she were at a buffet. That's where she ate her first endive."

"One of the most important parts, I think, is get-ting children excited about food," says Cosentino. "It promotes more questions, more interests in different things on a regular basis . . . you make them more inquisitive. My son Easton has been going to the farm-ers' markets since the day he was born; he's been a part of that system ever since the beginning. It's been a pretty interesting dynamic for us. He knows what things are in season, he waits for certain things, and he gets really excited about it. He loves apples, but apples are done for him right now because berries are in season. He looks forward to asparagus, but then he's done with it after a while."

Cathal Armstrong, chef and co-owner of Res-taurant Eve; Eamonn's, a Dublin Chipper; and The Majestic in Alexandria, Virginia, grows vegetables in a tiny greenhouse at home. "The kids participating in that element makes them a little more interested in trying foods they wouldn't normally eat because they see them," he says. "They participate in planting the seeds, the excitement of having the first sprouts come out of the ground, seeing the fruit come up. That makes them considerably more interested in trying something than if you go to the grocery store and pick up a bunch of radishes—most kids won't eat them. If the kids plant radishes, they produce fruit within a few weeks." Kravich says she planted seeds in her garden with her kids. They watched them sprout and grow, which "connected them to the earth and was symbolic to how they looked at life and creation," she explains.

Chefs all agree the preschool years are not a time to narrow their children's diet. The goal with pre-schoolers is to get them to continue to eat broadly. Vegetables, it's no surprise, are the foods most often rejected by this age group. When I asked Chef Linton Hopkins why his children love vegetables, he said, "I don't overcook vegetables. Overcooked, bland food, no one likes, especially kids." In the wintertime, he regularly cooks greens in a skillet for his kids. "I've found the kids really don't love the real slow-braised-style green, so we get the skillet really hot and add a little bit of fat and just hit it real hard in the pan, and it gets bright with a little acid—sometimes that's a pepper vinegar we have. If it's bright, fresh food, regardless of what kind it is, I think kids are going to enjoy it. The one thing I find with home cooks—I don't think they season enough to make a dish sharpened and focused to where it makes your mouth water."

It's not surprising, given hectic lifestyles and fussy children, that home cooks tend to revert back to the handful of recipes they know well and cook them repeatedly. Chefs, though, don't have limited menus and tend to cook creatively and experimentally. Diane Forley and Michael Otsuka, chefs and owners of Flourish Bakery in Scarsdale, have a strategy where they only bring foods into the house that they love to eat, or want to eat. They prepare foods from scratch and make sure that there's a range in terms of nutritional value. They believe food should taste good, and they prepare foods that they, themselves, want to eat. But then the kids lead them from there. There's a basis from which they start, but the developing likes and dislikes of the kids require them to simplify, eliminate, and adjust the meals and menus a bit as they go.

The menus in Cardoz's house were always mixed. "We wouldn't do the same thing every day," he says. "I just wanted them to be used to a lot of flavors. . . . The food always had some amount of spice in there or herbs in there. You know, lots of salt is bad for kids, but there would be some amount of salt in there too, just so that they understood what it was. . . . I did not do anything that was not recognizable, that was not familiar to them, like, there wouldn't be snails or chicken feet or tripe, things like that that kids don't like."

You can also entice kids by the way you describe a particular food or dish. Hopkins says, "A lot of times my wife will say, 'Kids, this is my famous turkey chili,' and they're like, 'Wow! Famous turkey chili!' You know, we'll describe a dish like that, and they want to be a part of the famous turkey chili!" Chefs agree that children have to see you enjoy food, too. If they see you enjoying something, they want to know what it is.

Chefs use a lot of patience with their children in regard to food. "It's very easy to say he's not eating anything, I'm just going to give him mac and cheese from a box," says Cardoz. "Instead, we've made mac and cheese from scratch. My son, when he was five, would ask me to make a five-cheese omelette for him for breakfast . . . and he was involved in grating the cheese, mixing the cheese, cracking the eggs. Yes, there was a mess in the kitchen and he cracked the eggs, but it was his omelette so he wanted to eat it."

Culture, History, and Family

Children at this age are highly impressionable; they will take the aromas of the foods we cook most often deep into their psyche. They create robust memories of what they see and do at this age. Cardoz says it was important for him when cooking with his children to always connect food with stories of how he grew up, "so there was some sense of culture and history and family with everything we did. I would tell them, 'My father would love to eat steak with potatoes,' and I would make those potatoes for them."

Curto-Randazzo says, "Probably the most popular dish among all of my kids is chicken cutlets—the chicken, thin, with seasoned bread crumbs, and I panfry it . . . then put a little lemon on it. It's something my grandmother would make, too. It's great the next day in the refrigerator. It's a very Italian thing to do, have chicken cutlets around." She mostly cooks Italian food at home because "that is my upbringing and my husband's upbringing, too . . . so there's always the Italian theme going on. . . . That was my comfort food. I'll make escarole soup with the little meatballs and white beans, homemade chicken soup with some pasta, or pasta with lentils."

Cookbook author and chef Peter Berley says that his children appreciated having had specially made lunches, like sandwiches made with good bread and nori rolls with brown rice. "They both say now, "These were the foods you made, that we loved, and we did feel really different and special." Cosentino's son, Easton, asks to go to a place they frequent together that he refers to as their "special noodle place." His son also loves cooking shabu shabu at Korean restaurants. Cosentino says eating foods from different cultures fosters curiosity about those cultures and makes learning interesting. He says, "History, food, and culture are not just about stuffing food into your stomach to get energy—there's more to it. History is behind everything."

Sortun sometimes makes meals fun by serving them away from the kitchen, at the coffee table where Siena, her daughter, is playing, "So that I can coax her out slowly, so that it doesn't seem like dinner is a punishment," she says. "Changing it around really helps me. Sometimes to make it fun we'll have breakfast in her tent in her room. . . . She's still kind of playing, but I'm getting her to focus on eating. I think there are a lot of distractions, and kids will play and think that eating is boring."

Cooking Strategies for Busy Families

For working parents and families who are really busy, it's good to have a perspective on what's important and a strategy for putting meals together. Making batches of foods and freezing portions can make dinner much easier. Meatballs, soups, and sauces can easily be frozen, as can cooked beans, fresh pasta, and cooked rice. Berley says his and his wife's schedules were always chaotic and unpredictable because they were both freelancing. He was working in restaurants and catering when his children were young. "Sitting down to eat was more important than cooking together . . . simply because I wasn't around—I was working a lot. . . . It didn't always work that we could cook dinner together. What I would do a lot of times is tell my wife what to start cooking—I would coordinate with her, like, why don't you start this [put the rice up for example], and I'd come home and finish up dinner real quick, and we'd sit down to eat. My real desire was to get them to eat as well as possible at home, as often as possible with us."

Sortun's strategy is to prepare a week's worth of food basics when home on the weekend. "I'll pick one day where I'll cook a few days' worth of meals—I make three or four meals," she says. "I'll make soup, I'll make chicken salad, I'll make a grain, and a chickpea and quinoa salad. That way there's stuff for lunch and dinner . . . there's always something to start from, so they can have a good balanced meal. My husband is good at cooking too, so I never have to worry, but it's a time issue. Trying to get them fed by a certain time can be a challenge. It makes it easier for them for the week when I'm not there for dinner—I'm usually working when they are having dinner. That way I know they are getting something good for dinner while I'm away."

Most chefs when cooking at home make only one meal—the family meal that everyone will eat. It happens in different ways at different chefs' homes. Some chefs plate the meals, others put food out and children and adults serve themselves from a dish, family style. For dinner, Blue Ribbon restaurants executive chef/co-owner Eric Bromberg and Armstrong both make a protein, a starch, and a vegetable,

"We have said from the beginning, our family meal is a family meal. So we really don't create special meals based on individual likes and dislikes. My children get input. . . . We'll talk about it ahead of time; when we go to the farmers' market on a certain day, we'll give them some money and they'll pick some things, so they're proud to bring those vegetables that they bought. And I think that's a great way to include them in the choices."

—Linton Hopkins, executive chef at Restaurant Eugene in Atlanta

and everyone chooses the foods they would like to eat. Sortun creates a design on the plate with the food, like bridges and tunnels and that sort of thing.

Eating Preferences— How to Cook for a Preschooler

"What we do is introduce a flavorful dish that is something they are going to be more familiar with, like pizza," says Armstrong. "We'll make it ourselves. From that platform, you can start to build ingredients like garlic and olive oil and basil and start to get more aggressive with flavors. You have to start with a foundation that kids understand." Cardoz agrees: "It's easier to put something in with something they already like. Some kids love shrimp—you can easily get kids to eat shrimp with rice if they don't like rice. Putting a dish together, I would never put all the strange things together, because I know my kids are going to be afraid of it." Curto-Randazzo adds, "If you put something on the table they really do like, you have a greater possibility of getting them to try something they might not."

ANDREA CURTO-RANDAZZO and her husband, **FRANK RANDAZZO,** are executive chefs of the Water Club in Miami. Previously, at Wish restaurant in Miami, Curto-Randazzo was named one of *Food & Wine*'s Ten Best Chefs. Randazzo was a contestant on *Top Chef*. They have three daughters, Isabella, Gia, and Lilli. Curto-Randazzo says, "I do want my kids to appreciate food because it's a beautiful thing, it's what I do, it's a big part of me. As chefs, my husband and I want them to appreciate all kinds of foods. And I always stress trying new things. For me, the person who got me to try new things was my grandfather. I'm sure by five or six, I was eating everything. He had me try pigs' feet, tripe, whatever. It was because he was my buddy, I wanted to be with him and be like him; so every time he gave me something new to try, I was all about it."

Lots of children who are three to five years old dislike spice, but Cody sometimes goes full force at something surprising like Dijon mustard and other times can't handle something as simple as herbs in eggs. Sometimes he says it smells funny, and it's a bigger challenge to convince him to take a bite. Cardoz advises parents to stay the course and be patient, and for his children he turned to more traditional family foods: "Which kid doesn't like meatballs?"

For other chefs, talking about ingredients and how they go together becomes important. To make his food flavorful and palatable for Zen, St. Petersburg chef Zack Gross uses a particular brand of smoked bacon: "For me, Nueske's bacon . . . that's something I don't skimp on. It adds so much to the dish. I love to have that wafting smell. Just to have that smell—smoky bacon—coming out of my oven first thing in the morning."

We learned from Bromberg to put mushrooms under the skin when roasting a chicken, and it is true, in our house, like his, a roast chicken will always go over well. For Tampa chef B. T. Nguyen, raw carrots, celery, and broccoli are staples. "Those are the three vegetables my son, James, loves, that I pack for him and have in the refrigerator all the time so he can snack on them."

Berley wasn't so concerned with teaching his kids about cooking or ingredients, "I was more concerned that they just enjoyed what they were eating—that was my main concern. I wanted them to have a good feeling and develop an attachment to eating real food. And, if they could develop that, then I figured if they got curious, the more they got curious, the more they'd want to know—and that's what happened."

For children who prefer pasta dinners, Berley suggests using semolina pasta, which is more nutritious because it has "a higher protein than pasta made from, say, a basic wheat bread flour." Whole grain durum wheat pasta, which is the whole durum wheat made as pasta, is another option. When you get whole wheat pasta from Italy, that's what you are

> **"There's got to be something they like that they can hang their hat on and say, 'Okay, I get it.' "**
>
> —Floyd Cardoz, New York City chef

getting. Berley suggests, "You can eat pasta with beans or meats and fishes and get even more nutrition in there."

"Yucky," "I Don't Like It," "I'm Full," and How to Change the Game

We do hear lots of "I'm not hungry" from Cody just as it's time for dinner, or at the table, things are frequently called "yucky" and "icky." Lots of kids will reject anything green, regardless of whether they consider the food to be otherwise palatable. With this age group, it's important to distinguish what is, in fact, about the food and what is about something else—like Cody's wanting control or feeling moody. Control issues around food are big at this age, instructs Cynthia Epps, a Los Angeles infant-feeding specialist. Not only do kids like to sort food so they themselves can control what they are eating, but they want to test the kind of control they can exert at mealtimes. All kids will experience this in some form or other. For some it is a quick and passing phase; for others it can be a prolonged and disruptive period of time.

How much we allow Cody at this age the independence of declaring he is or is not hungry has been a big question for us. The downside of letting the meal end when Cody says "he's full" is that sometimes he eats only a few bites of his meal and can get cranky from hunger later. Sortun says, "They know when they are full and when they have had enough. We are not sticklers for that kind of stuff as long as she's had a balanced meal." Nguyen sums it up when she says, "You have to give them the freedom to choose, but at the same time you have to focus them, expose

them." Gross keeps it all in perspective. He says, "I believe they have to make their own decisions. You try to teach them what you believe, but you can't fully make 'em do it. That's what I've realized. It's not worth getting upset about either. There's not enough time I spend with my daughter to want to be upset because she didn't want to eat something that I made for her." We would all be a lot happier if we relaxed a bit and had some fun.

Practically half of preschoolers aren't consistently hungry at mealtimes. One in four frequently refuses to eat; one in five asks for particular foods and then won't necessarily eat them. Statistics also show that half of all preschoolers try to end a meal after only a few bites. Cody has learned and frequently uses the phrase "I'm full," which we take to mean he's not engaged and we need to pay more attention to him during meals. At four years old, Cody went through a phase where he would *always* say, "I don't like it" when he first sat down—to everything. Giving him ways to participate helped, like letting him grate a little Parmesan cheese over his risotto or grind a bit of pepper into his stew. It's enough of a distraction for him to change the topic, and he forgets the fuss and eats.

Children at this age also begin to use language purposefully, and it creates tricky situations. They start to construct stories and learn catchphrases in order not to eat. Cody says with conviction about not eating his preschool packed lunch, "I was saving it for later." At home, when he says he's not hungry before mealtimes, I offer him an alternate truthful scenario, like suggesting he may not want to eat

CHRIS COSENTINO is the executive chef for Incanto, his San Francisco restaurant. Also, he is cocreator of Boccalone (www.boccalone.com), an artisanal salumeria, or cured-meat shop, also in San Francisco. Cosentino has a strong commitment to sustainable principles and humanely raised meats and is an avid researcher of ancient cooking techniques and culinary lore. He gained national acclaim as a leading proponent of offal cookery—cooking every part of an animal. The practice stems from a belief that no part of an animal slaughtered for food should go to waste.

Cosentino was raised by a single mom, but they lived close to his grandparents and all shared a weekly Sunday dinner. He firmly believes in the importance of that social family time. Of his son, Easton, he proudly says he can tell if strawberries are "too watery" or if the asparagus is not in peak season. "He always hangs around with the cooks in the restaurant; it's created a very interesting dynamic of taste and palate." Cosentino believes the most important thing is to be honest with kids, not to trick or lie to them to get them to try something. "It may not be the result you want right then and there, but the long-term result will be better."

Chef Chris Cosentino : NANCY NEIL

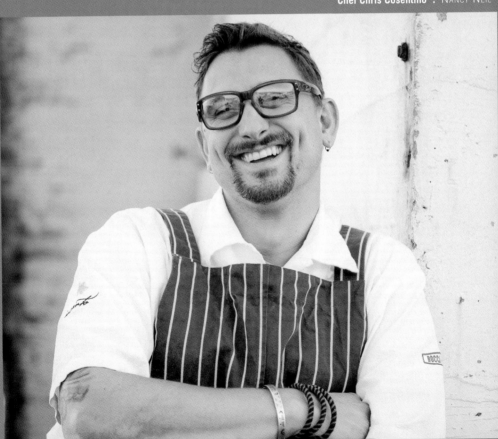

"My three-year-old is interested in beans from the vine—cooking them and eating them. We poach them and keep them crunchy, or sometimes we overcook them and make them mushy. He likes to play with them. So he's learning about how they can be different depending on how they're prepared."

—Alejandro Alcocer, New York City chef

because he would like to play instead. I know then that I need to make the meal a bit more fun to help engage him, and I propose a fun game we can play after eating.

Epps says that at meals "the most important thing you do is to not put anything in front of them at all." She explains that children's psychological boundary is the space right in front of them, at their fingertips, and that's the space they want to control. So it's better to serve food family style in the center of the table rather than putting the food directly on everyone's plate. Then, if they see you taking a serving of something and enjoying it, it will pique their curiosity and they're more likely to try it themselves, because it's their own idea to take some. "So set the food on a plate and only bring out the two things you want them to eat—set it down out of their reach," says Epps. "Sit down next to them and say, for example, 'we are having chicken and we are having asparagus.' Pick up a piece of chicken and start to eat and say, 'How was preschool today, did you see the clouds, it's raining outside?'—in other words, talk off topic."

Bromberg didn't worry too much about times when his children would go through phases, because they ate well most of the time. Nor is he overly concerned about the order of dishes. If his children are excited to eat a scoop of ice cream when they first sit down and doing so allows them to eat their broccoli and chicken after, then he's fine with that. "My wife and I both are of the 'clear your plate' generation," says Bromberg. "And that didn't really serve us well. We thought a different approach would be more successful, so we let them eat at the pace they're comfortable with and

try and give them options at mealtime. Yeah, we had challenging times; at one point our daughter only ate blueberries. I'm not kidding! She ate a pint of blueberries a day and nothing else."

Beginning to Cook

"What I did at three or four years old to get them involved in food was to cook with them," explains Cardoz. "I would sit them on the counter and make it so that it was fun. Make it so that they were involved. I would do things that were kid friendly. We'd make homemade chicken nuggets. . . . They like sushi, so we made sushi together. We've made meatballs together. We've made burgers together. We've made pasta sauce together. We've done everything."

Cooking is a wonderful activity for children of all ages, and all the chefs I spoke with cook with their kids at this age. Now, most children can measure, pour, and stir. An example of how savvy some chefs' children are in the kitchen at this age comes from Alejandro Alcocer, who says, "My five-year-old can cook pasta, roast tomatoes, and make a sauce. We have an electric induction stove, so he can't burn himself unless he touches the bottom of the pan. He's very careful when he lifts out the basket from the hot water. He mashes his roasted tomatoes and puts them on his pasta. He says 'I'm cooking!' It makes him a very confident little boy and gives him a sense of independence to know he can feed himself."

Marc Murphy's daughter uses a special stepstool called a Learning Tower so she can cook with him and be safe and comfortable at counter height. He taught

Make rules clear and be "patient and persistent," says Chef Cathal Armstrong. Rules do work better if you stick to them and aren't mean about it. Also, the earlier you set them the better. Of course kids will test the boundaries, but I find a lighthearted approach to enforcing them works. I continue playing a game with Cody where bites have vehicle sounds. Once, Cody cleverly replied to the car-sound bite, "Tunnel's closed for construction"; my reply was, "They're on a lunch break," and he took the bite.

•• **Keep trying.** Studies show that you may have to offer preschoolers a new food ten to sixteen times before they'll accept it.

•• **Children must taste the food before rejecting it.** Chef Floyd Cardoz says, "If you don't like it that's fine, but you have to taste it." This, actually, is not as hard as it sounds if you set the rule and stick to it.

•• **Relax and make meals fun.** Make mealtimes about eating and socializing, and don't be afraid to have fun. You can be silly and still have good table manners! No playing with food—throwing food or spitting food included—but that doesn't mean you can't be playful. Try a game to engage your child (or distract him if he's acting up): "Open your mouth and close your eyes and I will give you a big surprise! Guess what bite it is: zucchini bite? Rice bite?"

•• **Dipping.** I put toast rectangles alongside Cody's soup for dipping. I can convince him to taste the soup by dipping the bread in or even floating pieces of bread in the bowl of soup that he can fish out with his spoon. You can also count the bread bites. Counting is big fun in our house.

•• **Mixing bites.** A new food goes over better in the company of a familiar food. Some foods together are just so much better than separately.

•• **Try a different preparation.** Foods that are rejected may be enjoyed if prepared differently. Foods that are strongly disliked shouldn't be pushed. Chef Diane Forley says, "I don't sneak things in because she knows!"

•• **Talk about flavors.** Help your kids learn which foods are salty or bitter or rich or sour to build a vocabulary around food. I know Cody really enjoys the authority of tasting and declaring something is sour.

•• **Make only one meal.** No one wants to be a short-order cook in her own home. Make only one family meal and let everyone eat the parts of it that appeal to her.

•• **Get saucy.** Like dipping, sauces can be an incentive to eat. Chefs try different sauces with foods and let their children make their own combinations. We dip chips in yogurt and carrots in yogurt mixed with tahini. We also try mixing in herbs and spices.

Serve small portions on small plates. "I use miniature cups for Siena so she can finish the whole cup," says Chef Ana Sortun. "We want her to drink water, and we have better success if she's not overwhelmed by the size of the cup. It looks like she can accomplish something. She can handle the amount of water that's in that cup. And I keep filling up the cup. Those kinds of things work. I never give her a huge plate of food."

Use cool plates and spoons worth mentioning. Cody particularly likes a colorful Asian soupspoon from my mother. He will eat more because he likes the spoon.

Eat with friends whose kids eat well. Cody was a model participant in this program, and many kids would eat double their normal four-bite intake in his company. Of course, it goes the other way too, as we are learning now at four and a half.

Children must sit down at the table and stay at the table while the meal is going on. "You don't need to eat, but you need to sit" works well for us to get Cody to the table; talking about things he's interested in helps keep him there.

Don't give up. "It's really easy to give up and say, 'Okay, here are chicken fingers'. And every once in a while you do that because of the exhaustion, but you have to keep at it and keep on them because there are going to be chicken fingers forever," says Chef Andrea Curto-Randazzo.

Grow a garden. "Let the kids participate in growing their own food, and they tend to be much more excited about trying it," says Chef Cathal Armstrong.

Talk to your child's preschool teacher. Suggest starting a small vegetable garden in pots at school. Also, ask the teacher to help the kids eat lunch. Many children will not eat their lunch at preschools if, instead, they are allowed to play.

Don't reward with sweets and chocolates. Instead, reward and treat your children with activities and love.

Read books. Sally Kravich, a natural health expert, used to read *In the Night Kitchen* by Maurice Sendak to her children to inspire them to cook with her. Together they would make healthy versions of cakes and pies with fruits and nuts.

her to make an omelette. "She takes the fork, brings in the edges from all sides. She learns by doing. I teach her about heat. When the pan is hot, I have her hold her hand above it so she can feel the heat. She'll say to me, 'Daddy, that's hot. That's too grown-up for me to touch.' She looks at the knives and says, 'That's a grown-up knife. I can't use that.' She knows that I'm an adult and she's a child. She knows she's learning."

"I've created a little square over by the stove," says Gross. "I put things in bowls that Zen can dump in the pan, getting her excited about cooking. And she has more of an appreciation to eat things."

REASONS FEEDING A PRESCHOOLER MAY BE HARD

- They can be quick to dismantle something and eat only the part they want.

- They learn the word *yuck*, and it's an easy way to reject stuff.

- They are creatures of habit and create associative memories. If they've had candy or a treat at a store while shopping, they will want that same treat the next visit because they associate the two together. Although this is true of younger children also, at this age they are more outspoken and insistent.

- They love a colorful, crinkly package. For us, this meant a foray into the world of snack packages and trying to figure out moderation. Sometimes, group playdates can end up being snack fests because everyone generously shows up with a big bag to share and the kids overindulge.

- They want what their friends have. If they spot ice cream anywhere in the vicinity, they want one too, and at school they want the foods their friends have. "It is difficult at that time. It all depends on what their friends are eating and how often they hang out with their friends—and what their friends eat at home," says Floyd Cardoz.

- They are persistent and persuasive. Saying "no" repeatedly can be difficult.

- Getting food in their mouths is only half the battle. Preschoolers love to spit out food, let it fall out of their mouths, swing food around that is only partially in their mouths, and throw food. Also, I still fork feed Cody things to try. Sometimes, he's just as likely to spit it out.

- They know the word *treat*, and it can be difficult to ensure that they eat sugary foods in moderation.

CATHAL ARMSTRONG, a native Dubliner, was honored as one of *Food & Wine*'s Top Ten Best New Chefs in 2006. He was a nominee in 2007 for the James Beard Award Best Chef Mid-Atlantic for his four restaurants: Eve; The Tasting Room at Eve; Eamonn's: A Dublin Chipper; and The Majestic, in Alexandria, Virginia. He and his wife, Michelle, have two children, Eve and Eamonn. "I always get the kids involved in making the dinner, picking the herbs, peeling the garlic, chopping the garlic, and things like that—with a garlic crusher, not with a knife; they are not ready for knives yet. I think it's really important to be involved in the preparation of the meal and the cleanup of the meal because it develops good habits and good sensibilities in general," he says.

Cathal and Michelle Armstrong, daughter Eve, and son Eamonn : STACY ZARIN GOLDBERG

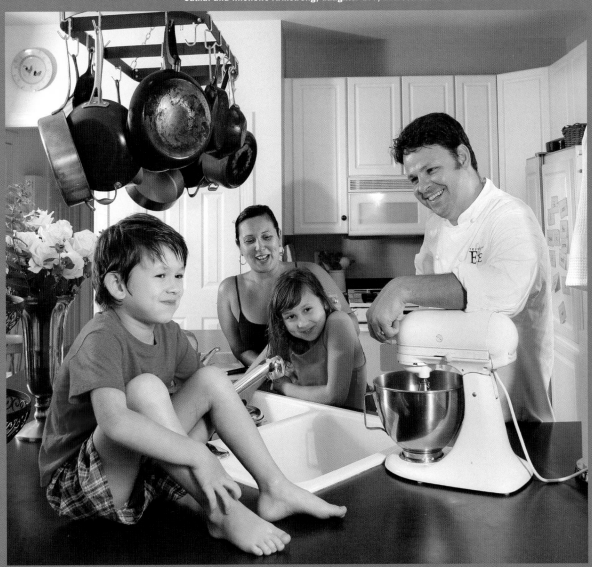

> "What's important, I think, is to keep the variety around Siena and get her involved in the cooking thing. Not to do it professionally, just as a skill to have, to feed herself well."
>
> —Ana Sortun, chef/owner of Oleana restaurant in Cambridge, Massachusetts

When chefs cook at home, they don't plan menus and make shopping lists. Instead, they cook spontaneously. "I'm a skilled chef—this is what I do. I would pick something up on the way home, bring something from the restaurant, and convert it into something else—it was very much on the fly," says Hopkins. Chefs know instinctively how the flavors of foods will go together, and, unlike most of us, can improvise meals. They use their senses along the way to make creative adjustments. They expose their children to the experimental way of cooking.

As a home cook, I don't have the same resources or know how to cook like chefs do, but, for Cody and me, cooking is a still a fun way to experiment and get creative, even if sometimes we make something that's not so good. We talk about being open to trying something new and it's okay if things don't go so well.

Armstrong's children "have little chef uniforms. They'll put them on and get involved in making bread and cakes and stuff. They love that kind of thing."

Lunch at School

"We talk about lunches. For instance, today I asked him what he wanted for lunch, and he told me he wanted a tamale, some raspberries, applesauce, and rice cake," says Cosentino, who says son Easton always eats his lunch.

I started talking with Cody, too, about lunch, but noticed when he attended a new preschool for the summer, when he was four, that his lunch would come home having been only nibbled at. Cody has always eaten his lunch, whether at home, at restaurants, with friends on lunch dates, or at his regular school. As it turned out, the children at his school who are finished with their lunch have free play, so, of course, Cody would rather play with his friends than sit by himself and eat lunch. I began to pack lunches that were simpler and quicker to eat. I think children in preschool are too young to be left to their own devices at school when it comes time for lunch. It's very stimulating for them to eat with all their friends, and they need some guidance about the importance of eating lunch.

I know that when Cody doesn't eat his lunch at school, he is hungry right when I pick him up, and any after-school plans get put on hold until he eats. I am usually caught off guard, and all I have are some simple snacks, when what he really needs is protein. It's too hard to pack a lunch and then bring a whole other meal for after school.

"I'll give her cold chicken cutlets to take to school. She'll eat it. Typically, we pack the lunch for her—turkey sandwiches are really popular, so I can't say we get too creative there. She'll eat the heck out of a turkey or peanut butter sandwich," Andrea Curto-Randazzo.

Notes about Foods and Health

Food stimulates the senses and provides sustenance, nourishment, and comfort. It should make you feel good; it should be adventurous but not gluttonous. Eating a variety of foods is key and so

ANA SORTUN opened Oleana, her Cambridge, Massachusetts restaurant in 2001. She also has a bakery and cafe called Sofra. The *New York Times* called her cooking "deeply inventive." In 2005 the James Beard Foundation named her Best Chef Northeast. She favors Mediterranean cooking—including lots of beans and purees. She published a cookbook, *Spice: Flavors of the Eastern Mediterranean*. Of her daughter Siena's eating she says, "Her mom's a chef and her dad's a farmer—there's a lot of variety all the time. She's really into the stuff my husband grows, and she eats stuff right out of the field, stuff that I think she's not going to like, like spicy greens. She knows where it comes from. That's a big part of it."

Ana Sortun, husband Chris Kurth, and daughter Siena : MICHAEL PIAZZA

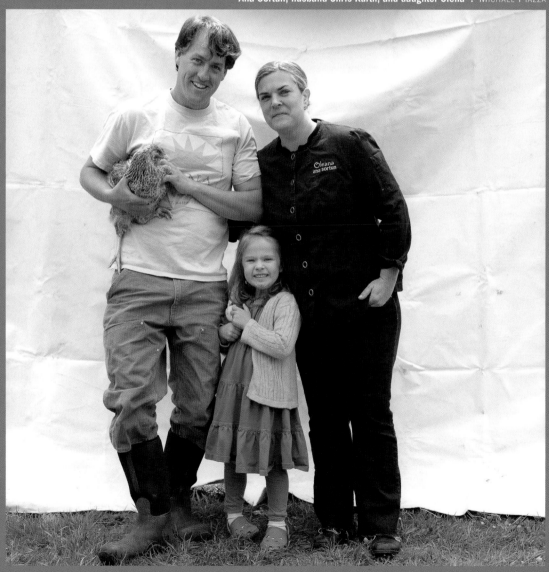

is moderation. I was once told that the best thing to teach your child was delayed gratification, and I would add moderation. I had kept Cody away from candy up until now, but at four I took him for a chocolate. It was actually a chocolate-covered salted caramel. We got a package or two from a special shop where we could sit outside on a bench under a tree. He watched me carefully unwrap the package, and I gave one to him and had one myself. We stared at each other, eating them slowly, bite by bite. They were so delicate and decadent that when we were done we just sat quietly for a moment, letting the flavor and the joy of it sink in. There are some things that are special and the experience of indulging in them is embraced. Foods that are decadent should be enjoyed consciously and those times acknowledged as special occasions.

What is health about at this age? Active four-year-olds need a surprising number of calories, and nutritionists say that eating a variety of foods is critical. For us, most of our food is homemade and moderate in its decadence, and it includes lots of vegetables and a good mix of whole grains. I admit to putting a pat of butter in our tomato sauce and an extra sprinkle of cheese on pasta. We forgo donut shops and candy from supermarkets and instead from time to time make our own cookies, cakes, and ice cream. We stay away from processed, overly sugary, overly salty foods. We do find ourselves occasionally buying a crinkly bag of something in a rush on our way to a playground playdate. Most chefs do, too. Paul Virant, executive chef at Vie restaurant in Chicago, says he didn't want his children to have to feel different from their friends

because of the foods they were eating. Likewise, I allow Cody a big, crinkly-bagged, relatively healthy snack from time to time so he can fit it. Also, Murphy suggests that having too strict a policy leads to sneaking overindulgences.

Epps believes that restricting sugary foods during the first twelve to fourteen months sets what she calls a "near sensory response," and "if you have laid down a solid foundation with not too much exposure to overly sugary foods, children then, when they have these [sugary] foods are going to be just like kids—they're gonna try them, they will dive into the cake like the other ones, but then, they will push away from the table and go off and play. They are able to self-limit. It doesn't get out of hand." She believes that without the early exposure to candy and other overly sweet foods as a preschooler "real, real, sweet food tastes too sweet."

I find this to be true for Cody. We go for ice cream after school on hot days from time to time, and we've even eaten decadent cookie ice-cream sandwiches and make cakes and other treats, but he never overindulges. Interesting to me is that while I know he relishes every last spoonful of chocolate ice cream, he doesn't ask for it more than once a month. Further, if he asks for a treat and I say no, he's okay with that.

Epps warns, "Taste buds can be influenced by exposure. . . . It's just brain chemistry." She explains that children who have too much early exposure to foods that are continuously sweet and overly sweet can be easily triggered into craving those foods. "They experience strong cravings and will salivate at seeing them in the hands of another child or in a shop window. That's not limited to just infancy, it has a lot to do with eating disorders," she explains.

It's unfortunate to have to mention that some foods that should be so healthy and wholesome end up with chemicals and pesticides that none of us want our children eating. Dr. Charles Bembrook, the chief scientist of the Organic Center (www.organic-center .org) says that for families to limit chemical pesticide exposure, they should eat certified organic produce at least for their favorite fruits and vegetables. In summertime soft fruits and berries are better purchased as organic; in the fall, apples. I rely on the environmental working group that has a great list of produce to be wary of eating because of a potentially high concentration of chemical pesticides. Conventionally grown apples and nectarines are at the top of their list. Their list also includes cherries, peaches, pears, raspberries, imported grapes, strawberries, bell peppers, celery, potatoes, and spinach. Fruits and vegetables least likely to be contaminated with chemical pesticides are bananas, mangos, pineapples, corn, onions, avocados, peas, and cauliflower. It's often thought that peeling fruit will eliminate the pesticides from those fruits, but the flesh of a peach with its soft skin is riddled with pesticides, which is why it often tops the list of produce to avoid unless it is organic. Also consider that peeling an apple will remove about a third of the apple's nutrients.

Kids this age don't know between white bread and wheat, and instead of making chicken soup with rice—à la our favorite Maurice Sendak book—we make chicken soup with barley.

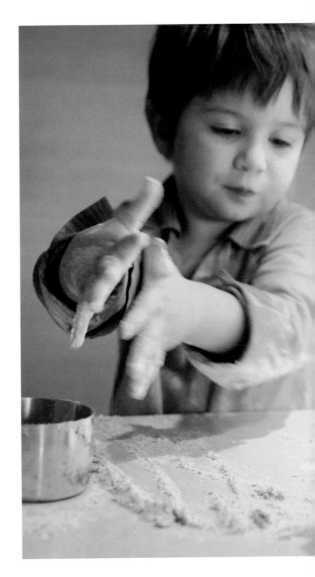

turkey meatballs with orecchiette pasta and tomato sauce

{ DIANE FORLEY }

Making meatballs is an act of love. They are always a bit time-consuming to craft, and they require a tender patience to make them just right. I make them for Cody because he gets excited for meatballs. They are the perfect thing to have in the freezer for a babysitter to make. On nights we go out, I like leaving Cody with something he knows is still homemade just for him. So I make a double batch. Sometimes I put them in a chicken soup with pasta, chard, and a good shaving of Parmesan cheese that Cody does himself at the table.

We also love them over pasta with sauce (see my recipe at right for tomato sauce). In general, the longer you cook tomato sauce, the more the acidity mellows out and the sweeter it becomes. Here, the sauce cooks for only 20 minutes, but a caramelized red onion creates that sweetness.

Note: Orecchiette pasta is a small shell-shaped pasta that holds the sauce like a little bowl would and makes a perfect mouthful.

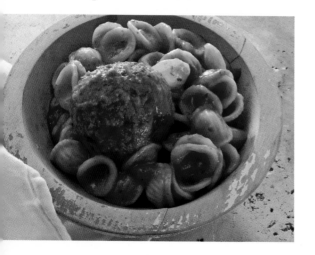

Meatballs:

3 tablespoons extra-virgin olive oil, divided

2 shallots, peeled and minced

3 cloves garlic, peeled and minced

Kosher salt and freshly ground black pepper

2 tablespoons water

1 tablespoon chopped fresh rosemary (or 1 teaspoon dried)

1 tablespoon chopped fresh oregano (or 1 teaspoon dried, crumbled)

½ teaspoon honey

2 tablespoons sour cream or plain yogurt

1 tablespoon Dijon mustard

1 egg, lightly beaten

2 teaspoons paprika, Hungarian sweet preferred

1 tablespoon dry mustard, preferably Colman's

1½ pounds ground turkey

¼ cup plus 1 tablespoon bread crumbs

Pasta:

1½ tablespoons salt

1 pound orecchiette pasta

Fanae's Quick Tomato Sauce:

1½ teaspoons olive oil

½ red onion, chopped

1 28-ounce can whole peeled tomatoes

½ cup tomato puree

1 tablespoon butter

8 basil leaves, optional

Salt and pepper

Pinch sugar, if needed

1. For the meatballs, heat a small skillet over medium heat and warm 2 tablespoons of the oil. Add the shallots, garlic, a big pinch of salt, and a good grinding of fresh black pepper and cook just until the oil begins to sizzle, about 2 minutes. Add 2 tablespoons water and cook until the shallots are soft and the pan dry, about 5 minutes; set aside to cool.

2. For the pasta, bring a large pot of water to a boil. Add 1½ tablespoons salt. When the water returns to a boil, add the pasta and cook until just tender. Drain.

3. In a large bowl, combine the shallot mixture, rosemary, oregano, honey, sour cream or yogurt, Dijon mustard, egg, paprika, and dry mustard and mix well. Add the turkey and season with ½ teaspoon salt and mix until combined. Add the bread crumbs and mix again until combined. With a rounded teaspoon or tablespoon, measure and scoop the mixture into small meatballs, the size of a quarter in diameter, onto a plate. You can also form by hand; keep your hands wet to prevent the meat from sticking to your hands.

4. In a medium saucepan over medium heat, add the remaining tablespoon of olive oil and brown the meatballs in batches, turning gingerly so as not to break them apart. Cook until browned on all sides; then remove them to a plate while making the sauce.

5. In the same saucepan, make the sauce. Add the olive oil or butter and the red onion and cook, stirring occasionally, until the onions are soft and lightly browned, about 5 minutes. Chop the tomatoes or squish with your hands into the saucepan with the juice from the can and the tomato puree. Stir to combine and add the meatballs back into the pan to continue cooking. Stir occasionally, being careful not to break the meatballs, and simmer for 10 minutes.

6. Add the butter to the tomato sauce. Turn off the heat and add the basil leaves; taste for seasoning and add salt and pepper and a pinch of sugar if necessary.

7. Divide the pasta into bowls; top with the meatballs and sauce.

Notes: The best way to freeze meatballs is to brown them first in the pan and freeze them half cooked. After spacing them out on a tray or plates so they are not touching, put the tray or plates in the freezer for an hour. Once set, the frozen meatballs can be placed in a freezer bag without clumping together and used as needed for up to one month. When ready to cook, add frozen to cook in the simmering sauce. An easier way to make meatballs is to turn the meat mixture out onto a long piece of plastic wrap and then form into a log. Unwrap and cut slices and form into meatballs.

boccalone sausage and beans

{ CHRIS COSENTINO }

SERVES 4

Chef Chris Cosentino has a shop in San Francisco, called Boccalone, that sells cured meats and sausages. This dish is especially good with the Italian sausage from his shop.

1 pound dried cannellini beans
Water to cover
3 quarts pork stock
6 cloves garlic, peeled and crushed, divided
1 whole carrot, peeled
1 whole fennel bulb, split
1 whole peeled onion
1 14½-ounce can plum tomatoes, chopped
1 tablespoon olive oil
1½ pounds Italian sausage links, cooked or uncooked
4–5 fresh sage leaves
Salt and freshly ground black pepper

1. Sort through the dry beans, removing any stones, then rinse under cold running water. Place beans in a large pot and cover by at least a couple of inches with cold water. Let soak for at least 4 hours or overnight. Alternatively, bring to a boil, cover, simmer for 5 minutes, then turn off heat and let rest covered for 1 hour.

2. Drain the beans and return to pot. Add pork stock, 2 of the garlic cloves, carrot, fennel, onion, and canned tomatoes. Bring to a simmer over medium heat and then lower the heat so that the beans are barely simmering and cook 1 to 2 hours, or until beans are just tender. Note that the fresher the beans, the shorter the cooking time. Remove from heat and let cool in cooking liquid. Remove the whole vegetables.

3. Heat olive oil in a large, heavy-bottomed skillet over medium heat. Add the sausage links and remaining crushed garlic cloves. Do not crowd the pan, or the sausage won't brown well. Once the sausage is brown, cut in half on the diagonal, add the sage leaves, let sizzle, then add the reserved beans in their cooking liquid, stirring occasionally until slightly thickened, about 5 minutes.

4. Season to taste with salt and pepper. Simmer a few minutes longer, stirring gently, until sausage is cooked through and the sauce has thickened. Be careful not to break up the beans.

Note: This recipe calls for preparing dried beans. However, you can skip steps 1 and 2 in the recipe by substituting 3 15-ounce cans of beans, rinsed and drained.

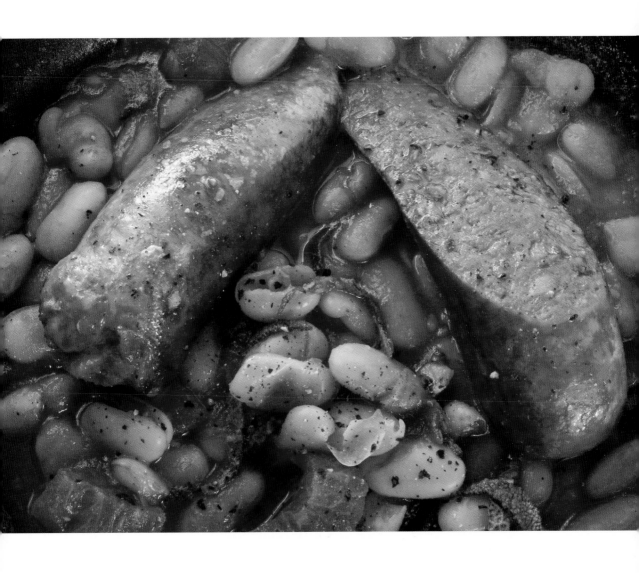

baby lamb chops

{ DIANE FORLEY }

SERVES 4-6

These are fast and easy to prepare for a quick dinner with children next to you in the kitchen. Chef Diane Forley recommends serving them with Ratatouille with Balsamic Vinegar, Honey, and Basil (page 55).

8 double lamb chops
Kosher salt and freshly ground black pepper
4 tablespoons olive oil

To cook the lamb, heat two large sauté pans over medium-high heat. Season lamb with salt and pepper. Add 2 tablespoons of the olive oil to each sauté pan and add the chops. Brown the lamb on all sides, turning every 2 to 3 minutes, about 7 minutes total for medium rare. Cut a small slice in the chop to check for doneness. Transfer to platter and allow to rest for about 5 minutes before serving.

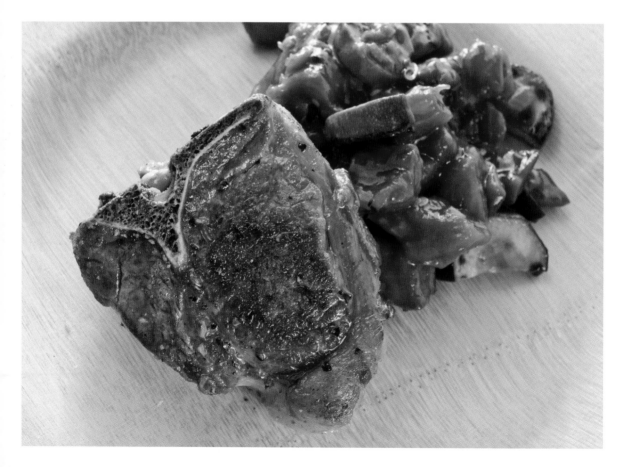

spiced beef sandwiches

{ CATHAL ARMSTRONG }

SERVES 4

The meat in this recipe marinates in spices all week in the fridge but is well worth the wait. A perfect early weekday dinner: warm sandwiches on whole wheat toast spread with the sauce left in the pan and horseradish. We had pickles on the side, and Cody couldn't decide whether he wanted his very last bite to be a sandwich bite or a pickle bite. After the last bite he suggested we lie down and take a nap on the couch, but we ended up playing at the table, trying to decide if his toy dinosaurs were meat eaters—and would've liked the sandwich meat—or plant eaters.

½ teaspoon ground cloves

½ teaspoon freshly ground black pepper

½ teaspoon ground allspice

½ teaspoon ground cinnamon

½ teaspoon ground mace

1 tablespoon brown sugar

2 tablespoons salt

2 teaspoons molasses

2 pounds boneless tied rib roast of beef

6 ounces Guinness beer

Water

Horseradish, optional

1. Mix all of the spices, sugar, and salt together. Add the molasses and rub the mixture all over the beef. Place in a nonreactive container in the refrigerator for 7 days. Every day, turn and rub the beef.

2. Place the beef in a pot and add Guinness and water to cover. Bring to a simmer and cook for about 3 hours until tender but not falling apart. Let cool in the cooking liquid. When cool, remove the beef and refrigerate until cold before serving.

3. Serve with wheat or pumpernickel bread. Horseradish can be added to taste.

delicate root vegetables

{ CATHAL ARMSTRONG }

SERVES 4

It's handy to have vegetables ready in the fridge to whip up quickly on a busy night. We do a lot of roasting of root vegetables in our house, but have found that preparing them this way gives the vegetables a nice, more subtle flavor. If you're getting your vegetables fresh from the farmers' market, you may not need to add the sugar.

4 baby carrots
4 baby turnips
4 baby parsnips
Water to cover
Salt
Sugar
1 teaspoon butter
Pepper

1. Peel and cut the root vegetables into even-size chunks. Place the carrots, turnips, and parsnips in separate small pots (they have different cooking times) and cover with water and season with salt. Add three parts sugar for each part salt to the water. Bring to a simmer.

2. When tender, drain and cool the vegetables by running cold water over them. Set aside in the refrigerator until ready to serve. This step can be done up to a day in advance.

3. In a small sauté pan, warm the root vegetables with a little butter. Season with salt and pepper.

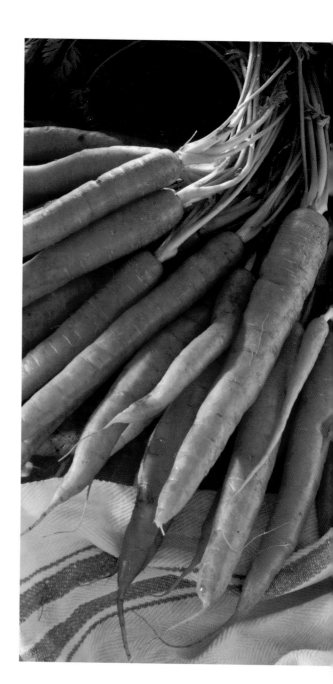

simple leafy greens

{ PETER BERLEY }

"From the time they were three years old, practically daily, they've been eating leafy green vegetables, hearty winter greens from the fall through the spring and lettuces in the summer," Chef Peter Berley says of his children. We eat these all the time at our house, too. Sometimes we eat them plain like this, and other times we add them to pasta or rice with some Parmesan cheese on top. They are great on spinach ravioli that has nothing else but a light sauce of chicken stock with a bit of butter.

1 pound winter or fall greens—chard, kale, and
    collard greens are all good choices
1 tablespoon olive oil
Salt and pepper

1. Bring a large pot of water to a boil. Wash and chop the greens, removing any tough stems. Add the greens to the water and cook until they are just a bit soft and bright green—all greens have different cooking times; chard is quick and kale takes a bit longer. They will shrink quite a bit. Don't overcook them; they should still be bright in color.

2. Once cooked, strain the greens, discarding the water.

3. Heat a large sauté pan; once hot, add the oil. When the oil is hot, add the greens and add salt. Stir and cook quickly until tender.

4. Add a grind or two of pepper, to your taste, and serve.

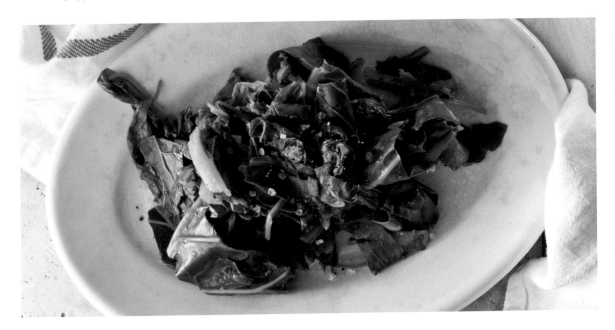

carrot salad with ginger

{ ANA SORTUN }

SERVES 4

Chef Ana Sortun makes this tasty salad for Siena for lunch. She suggests serving with pita bread cut into shapes, brushed with olive oil, and toasted. I made a batch to send one day to school for Cody and his friends to eat, and the bowl came back empty.

1 pound carrots, peeled and cut into 2-inch lengths
Water to cover
2 tablespoons extra-virgin olive oil
2 teaspoons white balsamic vinegar
1 teaspoon honey
¼ teaspoon ground ginger
Kosher salt to taste

1. Place carrots in a sauce pot with enough water to cover. Bring to a boil and simmer for about 20 to 25 minutes, until carrots are tender when squeezed with a pair of tongs.

2. Drain well and place carrots into a small mixing bowl.

3. Coarsely mash them with a whisk or a fork. Add the other ingredients and season with salt to taste.

curried chickpea salad

{ JOAN MCNAMARA }

SERVES 4

This dish is surprisingly good considering the ingredients are so simple, and it's a cinch to make. It's better to eat the same day, once you stir in the fresh herbs.

4 teaspoons best-quality olive oil
1 cup diced onions
½ teaspoon turmeric
½ teaspoon cumin
½ teaspoon coriander
¼ teaspoon cayenne pepper (optional)
2 15-ounce cans chickpeas, drained and rinsed
4 teaspoons lemon juice, or to taste
¼ teaspoon salt
Pepper to taste
2 tablespoons chopped fresh cilantro or parsley

1. Heat a sauté pan large enough to easily hold the beans over medium heat. When hot, add the oil to heat, then add the onion and sauté until deeply colored, about 6 to 8 minutes, stirring periodically.

2. Add the turmeric, cumin, coriander, and cayenne pepper, if using, and continue to sauté until the spices are aromatic and a bit toasted, about 3 minutes.

3. Add the chickpeas, lemon juice, salt, and pepper and cook for another 5 minutes to blend the flavors.

4. Remove from heat and cool. Store in the refrigerator, or mix in the fresh cilantro or parsley and serve immediately.

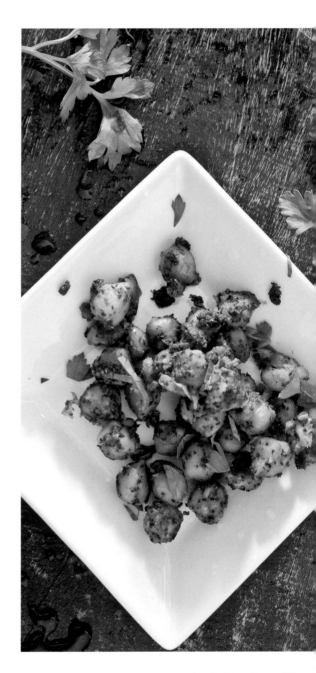

deviled eggs with tuna

{ ANA SORTUN }

Chef Ana Sortun suggests making this as part of a packed lunch along with Carrot Salad with Ginger (page 96). Assembled this way the tuna is milder tasting. For a treat use fresh tuna instead of canned.

½ cup minced celery

Large pinch curry powder

½ teaspoon paprika

1 6-ounce can water-packed tuna, drained, or 6 ounces fresh tuna

2 teaspoons extra-virgin olive oil

4 hard-boiled eggs, split in half lengthwise, with yolks removed and whites set aside

1 cup mayonnaise or half mayonnaise/half plain yogurt

Salt and pepper to taste

Cupcake wrappers for packing in a lunchbox (optional)

1. In a small sauté pan, sauté the celery, curry powder, paprika, and fresh tuna (if using) in olive oil for about 3 minutes, until the tuna is just cooked through. Cool, drain well, and chop by hand. If using canned tuna, just sauté the celery with curry and paprika in oil until the celery softens, then combine with the canned tuna in a bowl.

2. In a small mixing bowl, mash egg yolks with a fork. Stir in mayonnaise or mayonnaise/yogurt combination and tuna mixture. Season to taste with salt and pepper.

3. Fill centers of egg whites with a heaping spoon of tuna filling and serve or pack in cupcake wrappers for lunchboxes or picnics.

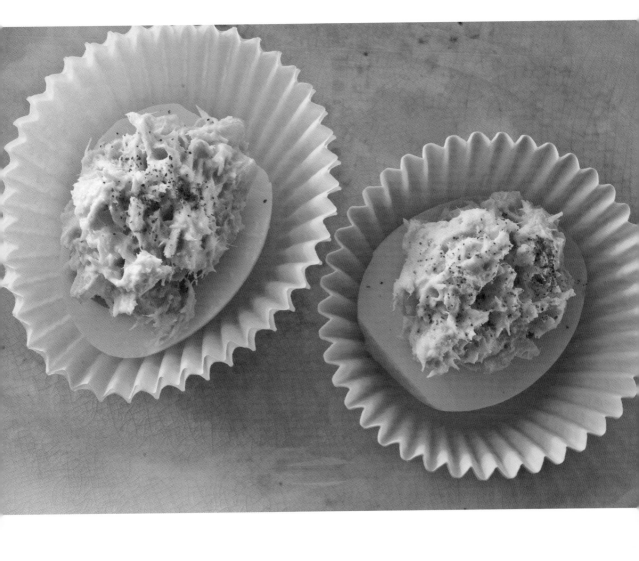

cannellini and yellow wax bean salad with shaved radish

{ CHRIS COSENTINO }

SERVES 4-6

The beans in this recipe soak overnight twice, which makes them especially tender and flavorful. In a pinch, add the olive oil when you first cook them, cook the beans a bit longer, and skip the second overnight soak, says Chef Chris Cosentino. When he makes this salad, it's beautiful with half rounds of onion and large chunks of radishes; here it calls for smaller kid-size bites.

Salad:

1½ cups dried cannellini beans

Water to cover

½ yellow onion

1 celery rib

1 carrot

Kosher salt and fresh black pepper

2 tablespoons extra-virgin olive oil

⅓ pound yellow wax beans, ends trimmed

¼ cup Zinfandel Vinaigrette (recipe below)

¼ red onion, sliced and chopped into small pieces

3 red radishes, chopped small

2 tablespoons chiffonade-cut basil leaves, preferably piccolo fino verde

Zinfandel Vinaigrette:

2 tablespoons Zinfandel vinegar, or good-quality red wine vinegar

¼ cup plus 2 tablespoons olive oil

2 tablespoons extra-virgin olive oil

Kosher salt

Freshly ground black pepper

Splash of lemon juice

1. Soak the dried cannellini beans in water for 4 hours or overnight in the refrigerator. Alternatively, place beans in a pot covered with 3 inches of water, bring to a boil, cover, and simmer for 5 minutes, then turn off heat and let rest, covered, for 1 hour.

2. Drain the beans, discarding the water, and place in a medium saucepan with whole peeled onion, celery, and carrot. Cover with cold water, bring to a simmer, and let cook until tender (about 2 hours). Remove the vegetables and season beans with salt and pepper and a good helping of extra-virgin olive oil. Let cool and set in the refrigerator overnight.

3. The next day, blanch yellow wax beans in a pot of salted boiling water until colorful but still crunchy (about 2 minutes) and shock in salted ice water to stop the cooking. Remove the beans from the ice water as soon as cold. (The beans will absorb water and lose flavor, so limit the time immersed in water if possible). Once cool chop beans into bite-size pieces.

4. For the vinaigrette, pour vinegar into a mixing bowl, then gradually whisk in the oils. Once the oils are incorporated, season with salt and fresh black pepper. To help with final balance, squeeze in a bit of lemon juice.

5. Strain the cannellini beans and place in a mixing bowl with the yellow wax beans, onion, and radishes.

Season with salt and pepper to taste; then dress with the desired amount of Zinfandel Vinaigrette. Sprinkle with basil leaves. Taste, adjust seasoning if needed, and serve.

Note: This recipe makes a good quantity of Zinfandel Vinaigrette. Keep any extra in the refrigerator for up to 1 week and use it to dress any cold vegetable or leafy green salads.

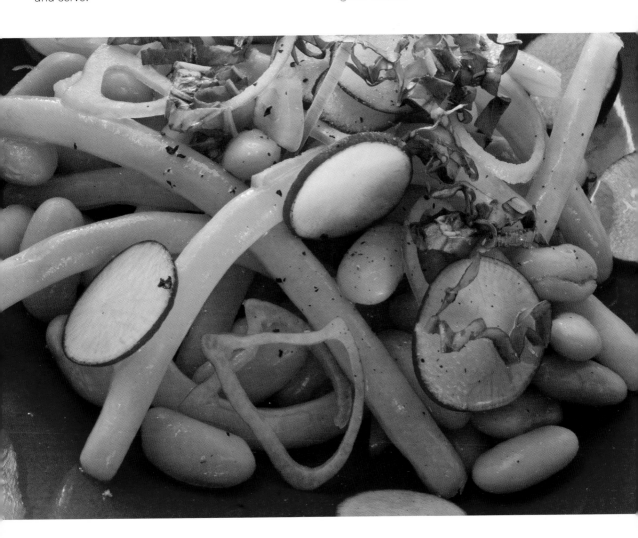

spaghetti pancakes

{ MARC MURPHY }

SERVES 4

This is a clever pancake version of macaroni and cheese. It's fun to make with kids, who always like noodles.

4 teaspoons salt
1 pound spaghetti
4 eggs
½ cup grated Parmesan cheese
½ cup grated pecorino cheese
½ cup grated Swiss cheese
4 slices American cheese, cut into quarters
Salt and pepper to taste
2 tablespoons olive oil

1. In a large pot bring 4 quarts of water to a boil. Add the salt, then add the pasta and cook until tender. Drain but don't rinse, and set aside to cool.

2. Meanwhile, mix the eggs and grated cheeses in a large bowl. Season with salt and pepper to taste and add the pasta.

3. Heat a large nonstick sauté pan on medium heat and add the oil. Put pancake-size messy scoopfuls of the spaghetti mixture in the pan and flatten each out. Lay the slices of American cheese on top and layer and flatten another smaller scoopful of the spaghetti mixture on top. When the bottom is golden brown, flip like a pancake and cook the other side, about 5 minutes a side, and serve warm.

yogurt panna cotta

{ BARBARA LYNCH }

SERVES 4

This is a simple luscious pudding made with gelatin, so it sets softly once chilled. Sometimes I pour it to set into old mismatched china teacups, but it's beautiful set into glasses with layers of fruit or compote or unmolded on a plate topped with berries. Cinnamon or other spices can be added, or it can also be served with chocolate sauce or caramel sauce.

¾ cup heavy cream
1 cup full-fat Greek-style yogurt, such as Fage Total
¼ cup sugar
¼ teaspoon pure vanilla extract
Kosher salt
1 teaspoons powdered gelatin
Fresh fruit or compote (optional)

1. In a medium saucepan, combine the cream, yogurt, sugar, vanilla extract, and a pinch of salt over medium heat just to dissolve the sugar.

2. Sprinkle the gelatin over ¼ cup cold water in a small saucepan and let it sit for 5 minutes to soften, then heat it over low heat until it becomes a clear liquid. Whisk this into the cream mixture and pour through a fine-mesh strainer.

3. Divide among 8 4- to 5-ounce ramekins or parfait glasses, cover with plastic wrap, and refrigerate until set, at least 4 hours, preferably overnight.

4. Serve the cold panna cottas garnished with fresh seasonal fruit or your favorite preserve, jam, or compote.

Note: These will hold, refrigerated and covered with plastic wrap, for 2 days.

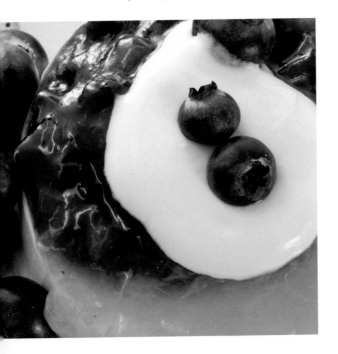

honey roasted nuts and fruit

{ MEGAN GARRELTS }

SERVES 4

We serve this to friends, and no matter how much we make, it's gone by the time they leave. Scrape into a container before it cools completely, because it does gets stuck to the pan or bowl pretty quick once it's cooled.

2 cups mixed nuts

1 teaspoon kosher salt

½ teaspoon freshly ground black pepper

Pinch cayenne pepper (optional, for kids who like a little spice)

⅓ cup honey

1½ teaspoons fresh chopped herbs: rosemary, sage, thyme

2 tablespoons golden raisins

2 tablespoons chopped dried figs

2 tablespoons chopped dried apricots

2 tablespoons chopped dates

1. Preheat oven to 350°F.

2. In a large bowl toss together the nuts, salt, peppers, and honey.

3. Lightly spray a baking sheet with nonstick cooking spray and spread the honey-coated nuts onto the sheet.

4. Bake the nuts for about 8 minutes, until they are evenly toasted, stirring and rotating the baking sheet within the oven during the baking time.

5. Once toasted, remove the nuts from the tray and transfer back into the large bowl. Toss the warm nuts together with the chopped herbs and dried fruit.

6. Allow the nuts to cool to room temperature and serve.

7. Place the nuts and fruit in an airtight container and store in the refrigerator for up to 2 weeks.

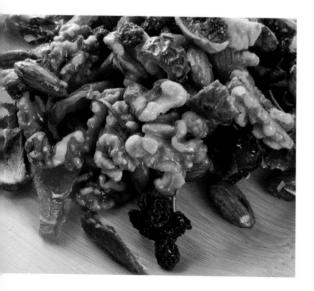

honey ginger ice cream

{ MEGAN GARRELTS }

YIELDS 1¼ QUARTS ICE CREAM, PLENTY FOR 4
SERVINGS PLUS EXTRAS

The ginger in the ice cream is subtle, and it makes a delicious and irresistible ice-cream flavor that leaves you wanting another scoop. This is great with Chef Megan Garrelts's Sugar Cookies (page 111) crumbled on top. She recommends serving the ice cream alongside her Warm Roasted Nectarines (page 112).

1 pint heavy cream

1 cup whole milk

½ cup brown sugar

½ cup Missouri honey (or *your* favorite local honey)

1½ teaspoons freshly grated gingerroot

6 egg yolks

1. In a large saucepan, combine cream, milk, brown sugar, honey, and freshly grated ginger. Warm over medium heat to infuse the honey and ginger into the cream.

2. Place the egg yolks in a stainless steel bowl and whisk to combine together.

3. Slowly whisk the hot cream into the egg yolks.

4. Strain the mixture through a fine sieve and chill over an ice bath.

5. Once the ice cream base is chilled, process in an ice-cream machine according to the manufacturer's instructions.

6. Serve and freeze any extra in an airtight container.

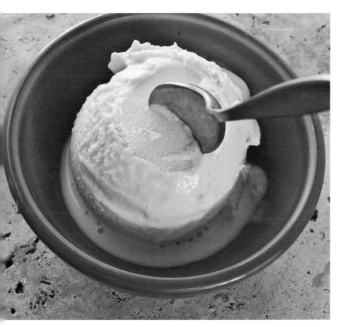

milk chocolate walnut ice cream

{ MEGAN GARRELTS }

YIELDS 1¼ QUARTS ICE CREAM

Making your own ice cream with friends over beats going to the store for ice-cream cones any day. Cody and his friends hover around the mixer and watch it churn before their eyes. This was the very first ice cream Cody and I made together, and it was the creamiest and most delicious chocolate ice cream I've had.

1 pint heavy cream
1 cup milk
1 cup sugar
6 egg yolks
6 ounces milk chocolate, melted
¼ cup toasted walnuts, coarsely ground

1. In a large saucepan combine cream, milk, and sugar. Warm over medium heat until tiny bubbles are visible along the edge of the milk, next to the side of the pan.

2. Place the egg yolks in a stainless steel bowl and whisk to combine.

3. Slowly whisk the hot cream into the egg yolks.

4. Whisk in the melted milk chocolate.

5. Strain the mixture through a fine sieve and chill over an ice bath.

6. Once chilled, process in an ice-cream machine according to the manufacturer's instructions.

7. Place the churned ice cream into a chilled bowl and fold in the toasted walnuts.

8. Serve and freeze any extra in an airtight container.

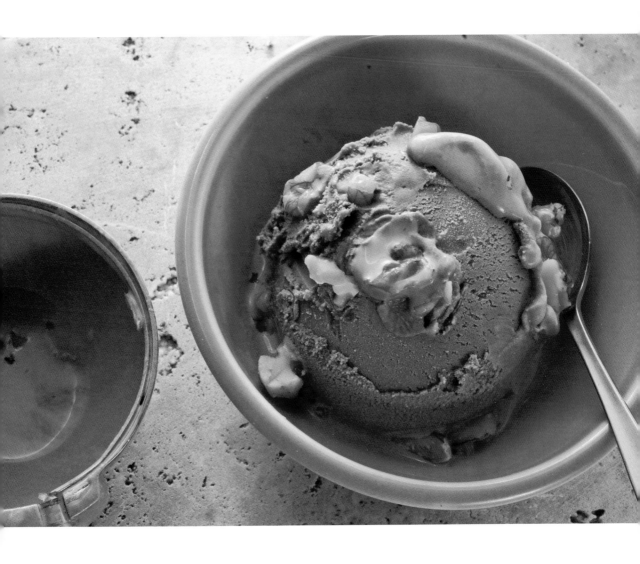

banana bread

{ MEGAN GARRELTS }

This makes a beautiful, high-rising loaf that is moist and flavorful on the inside and has a delicious crisp and crunchy crust. It's not the hearty or heavy banana bread with walnuts we're all familiar with. It is a special treat when served with Chef Megan Garrelts's Butterscotch Sauce (page 110).

2 cups flour

2 teaspoons baking powder

½ teaspoon salt

2 teaspoons cinnamon

½ teaspoon cardamom

½ teaspoon nutmeg

6 ounces unsalted butter at room temperature

1 cup sugar (plus some extra for coating the pan)

2 eggs at room temperature

2 teaspoons vanilla extract

1 cup milk

¼ cup buttermilk (see page 109)

Zest from 1 lemon

2 ripe bananas, mashed

1. Preheat oven to 350°F.

2. Sift the dry ingredients and set aside. Use whisk to make sure the dry ingredients are all mixed together, and you won't get an odd bite of baking soda in the bread.

3. Cream the butter and sugar; add eggs one at a time and vanilla.

4. Add the dry ingredients to the butter mixture alternately with the milk and buttermilk.

5. Mix in the lemon zest and mashed bananas—do not overmix.

6. Butter a loaf pan, then coat with sugar by adding a tablespoon or so to the pan and shaking it around. Pour the batter into the pan.

7. Bake in preheated oven until golden brown and firm to the touch and a toothpick comes out with crumbs, about 40 to 50 minutes.

Note: Creaming the butter and sugar gives baked goods a light airiness—they will be more delicate. Start with the butter soft, at room temperature, and beat with the eggs, also at room temperature, for several minutes, long enough to create tiny pockets of air. If you've forgotten to leave your butter out at room temperature to soften, you can use your microwave. Warm the butter on low in 10-second intervals and watch it carefully so it doesn't melt. To cream, place the softened butter into the bowl with the sugar. I use a wooden spoon to crush and mix the butter together with the sugar. In the end, the butter and sugar together should be fluffy.

······> Quick buttermilk can be easily made by mixing 1 cup milk with 1 tablespoon lemon juice or vinegar, which clabbers the milk. Let the mixture stand for 10 minutes, and it will thicken and clump up a bit. I actually like making pancakes and such with the lemon juice version; it gives them a brighter flavor. White vinegar (not cider vinegar) is flavor-neutral and clabbers the milk nicely without adding any fruit flavor. If you clabber your own milk, mix it alternatively with the milk so as not to also clabber the other milk called for in a recipe.

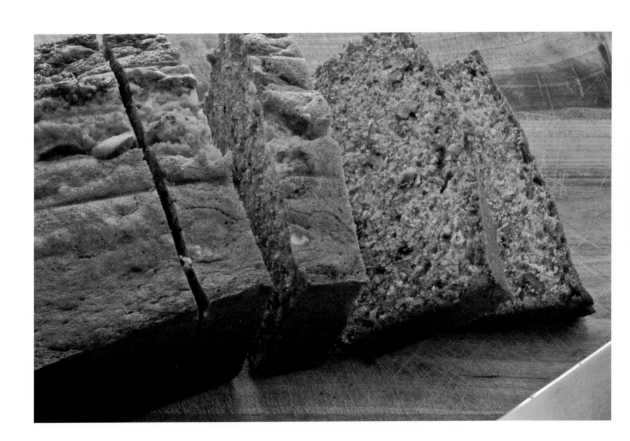

butterscotch sauce

{ MEGAN GARRELTS }

MAKES 1 CUP

Chef Megan Garrelts suggests drizzling this decadently over her Milk Chocolate Walnut Ice Cream (page 106) or spreading it on her Banana Bread (page 108).

1 cup brown sugar
1 cup unsalted butter, cut into pieces
½ cup cream
1 teaspoon lemon juice
½ teaspoon salt

1. In a saucepan, combine all the ingredients.

2. Whisking constantly, bring the mixture to a rapid boil and cook until it is a deep caramel color.

3. Strain through a fine sieve and keep warm.

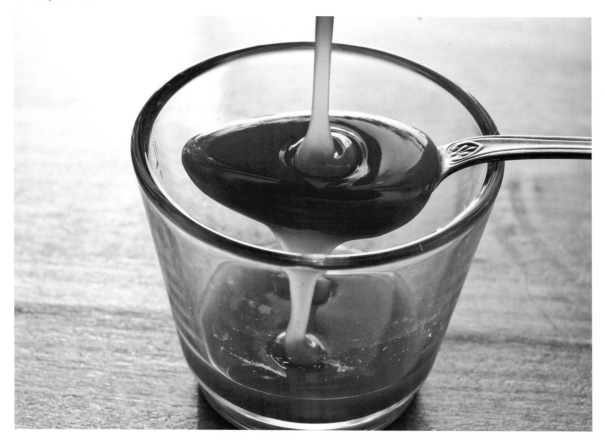

sugar cookies

{ MEGAN GARRELTS }

MAKES ABOUT 30 SMALL COOKIES

Delicate, with a hint of lemon and a satisfying crunch, these butter cookies are perfect. Make them by the sloppy tablespoon or use cookie cutters. Chef Megan Garrelts uses the dough to top her Summer Stone Fruit Cobbler with Crème Chantilly (page 114) and her Warm Roasted Nectarines (page 112).

2¼ cups flour
1½ teaspoons baking powder
1 teaspoon salt
2 sticks plus 2 tablespoons unsalted butter
1¼ cups sugar
1 teaspoon vanilla extract
½ lemon, juice and zest
1 egg

1. Sift the dry ingredients and set aside.

2. Cream the butter, sugar, vanilla, lemon juice, and lemon zest together.

3. Add the egg to the creamed mixture and mix well.

4. Add the dry ingredients in thirds, mixing each time.

5. Turn the dough out onto a piece of plastic wrap on the counter. Top with a second piece of plastic wrap and roll the dough into a flat disk about ¼-inch thick. Chill the dough until firm or store in the freezer for later use. (To store for making sugar cookies, gently roll dough in plastic wrap into an even log, about 2 inches in diameter, and store wrapped in aluminum foil or a re-sealable plastic bag in the freezer. Slice and bake straight out of the freezer, as needed, in a 350°F oven.) Bake until slightly golden, about 10 minutes.

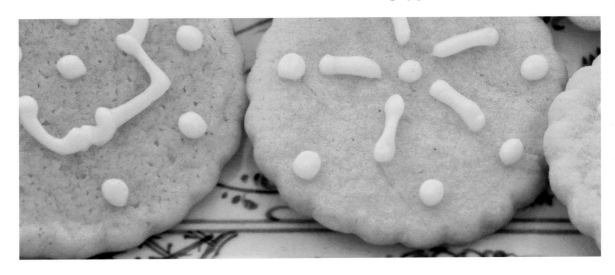

warm roasted nectarines

{ MEGAN GARRELTS }

These are great on their own, with a scoop of Honey Ginger Ice Cream (page 105) or with a dollop of yogurt in them. We use thick Greek-style yogurt. You can also drizzle some honey over the yogurt. Make them in the middle of the summer, when the fruit is deliciously ripe. As a special treat, make Sugar Cookies (page 111), crumble them, and sprinkle them over the top before serving.

4 nectarines
2 tablespoons brandy
¼ cup sweet white wine (or white grape juice)
¼ teaspoon vanilla extract
4 tablespoon sugar
1 tablespoon unsalted butter

1. Preheat oven to 350°F.

2. Split the nectarines in half and remove the pit.

3. Place the nectarines face up in a buttered roasting pan.

4. Mix the brandy, sweet wine, and vanilla together in a small bowl.

5. Pour the wine mixture over the nectarines (there will be some left over). Sprinkle the sugar over the fruit and dot with the butter.

6. Cover the pan with foil and roast the fruit in the oven until the fruit is tender but still holds its shape, about 30 minutes, depending on the ripeness of the nectarines.

7. Serve warm with desired accompaniments.

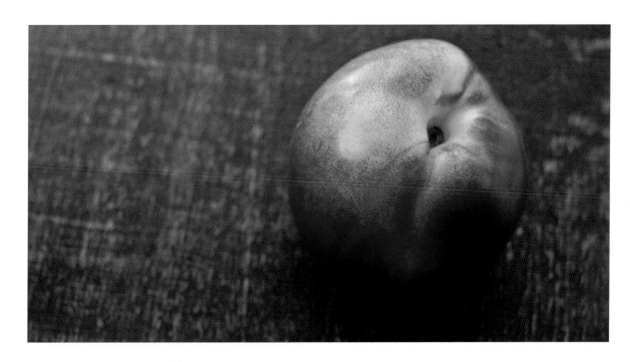

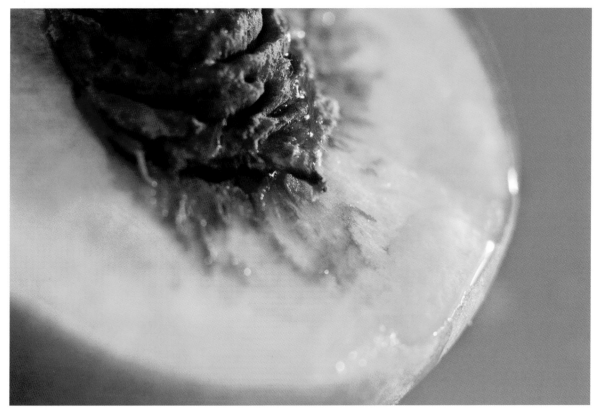

summer stone fruit cobbler with crème chantilly

{ MEGAN GARRELTS }

We make this in summer and bring it along for summer-evening picnics. Instead of making one big cobbler, we bake individual servings in cupcake wrappers in a muffin tin. This can also be made without the cookie crust for a simpler treat.

** *Note:* The Crème Chantilly can be made in advance and kept in the fridge for several days.**

Cobbler:

2 nectarines, cubed

2 peaches, cubed

1 cup assorted fresh berries, washed and hulled

2 tablespoons sugar (more if fruit is out of season
    and/or unripe)

¼ teaspoon cinnamon

¼ teaspoon cardamom

¼ teaspoon nutmeg

½ orange, juice and zest

¼ teaspoon freshly grated gingerroot

½ tablespoon cornstarch

½ batch sugar cookie dough (page 111)

¼ cup cream

¾ teaspoon ground cinnamon

2 tablespoons granulated sugar

Crème Chantilly:

1¼ cups heavy cream, well chilled

1 tablespoon confectioners' sugar, sifted

¾ teaspoon vanilla extract

1. Preheat the oven to 350°F.

2. To make the cobbler, combine the cut fruit in a large bowl and toss with sugar, spices, orange juice and zest, ginger, and cornstarch. Taste the mixture; you should be able to taste each flavor you added. Depending on the flavor of the fruit, you may need to add more spices, sugar, or cornstarch. Cornstarch should lightly coat each piece of fruit.

3. Mound the fruit mixture in a buttered and sugared cobbler dish or into cupcake wrappers in a muffin pan.

4. Cut chunks of sugar cookie dough and place on top of the fruit to cover most of the surface.

5. Mix the cinnamon and sugar. Brush cookie dough with cream and sprinkle cinnamon and sugar mixture on top.

6. Bake in the oven until the cookie dough is golden brown and the fruit begins to bubble, about 30 minutes.

7. Meanwhile, begin making the Crème Chantilly. Whip cream, sugar, and vanilla until stiff, then chill.

8. To serve, mound slices or spoonfuls of warm cobbler onto plates and top with Crème Chantilly.

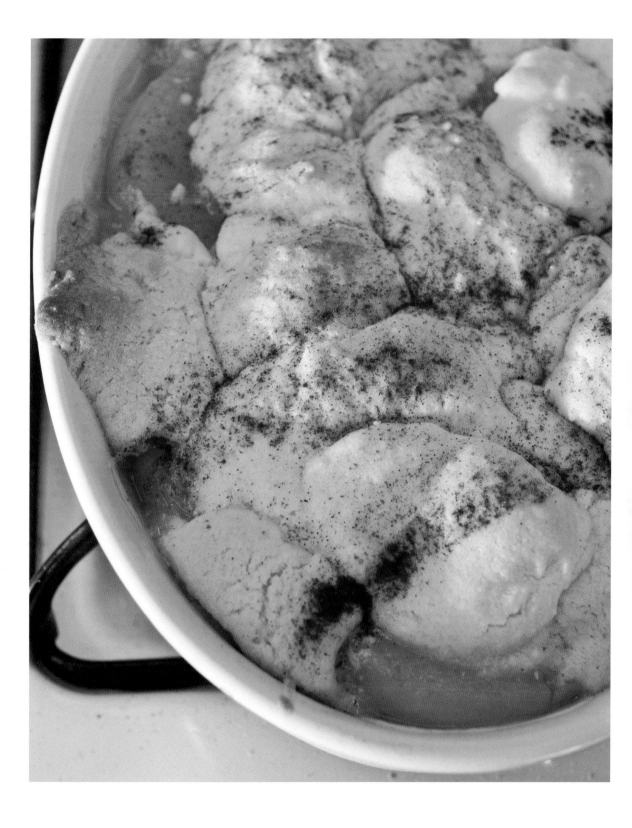

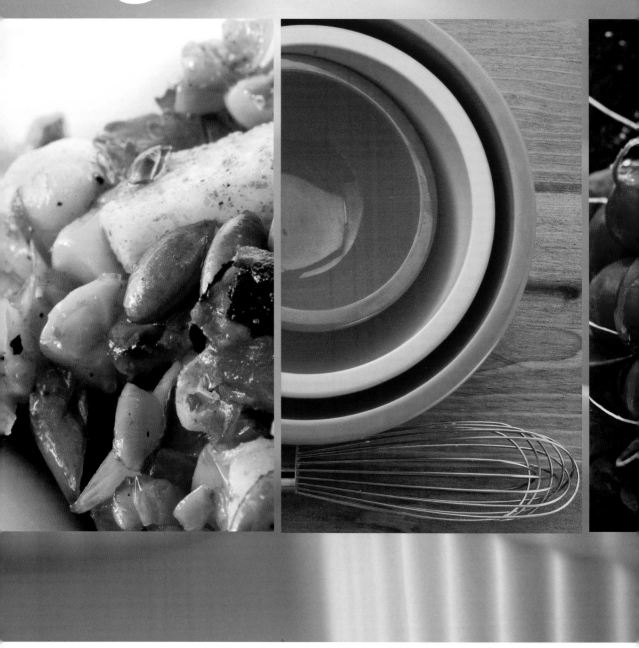

big kids

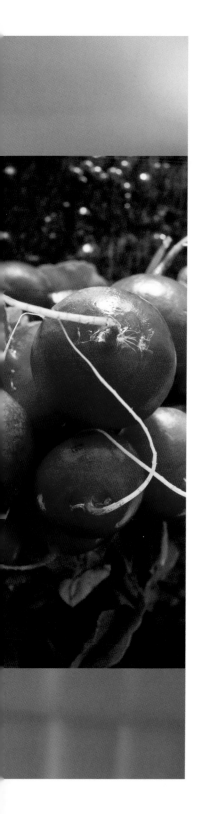

DEVELOPING
A PALATE

ages five to eight

Many children grow out of their fussy eating sometime between the ages of five and eight. It's common for younger children to resort to dietary quirks, such as separating foods so they don't touch on the plate and eating things like chicken and pasta without any sauce. Miami chef Andrea Curto-Randazzo says at this age her kids started to like dipping bread in olive oil and having sauce all over their pasta. She thinks children during this time "mature a little, they get a little more comfortable. . . . It's that age when they get a little more adventurous and start to enjoy food." She mentions that her daughter turned around at six years old and now loves fresh mozzarella, prosciutto, and salami. While kids are certainly a bit more adventurous at this age, some flavors will appeal to them more than others, and their willingness to try new foods may depend upon what you offer them and how you present it.

Introducing New Flavors

New York's Tabla restaurant executive chef and co-owner Floyd Cardoz says, "As children get older, it's all about making foods with contrast in flavors and texture. Not over-the-top bitter, over-the-top salty, or over-the-top spicy; you can't have all those things for kids." His children at this age began to eat things that, honestly, I don't even eat as an adult—like tripe. When they eat dim sum at a local Chinese restaurant, "they have a blast with chicken feet, snails, and clams. Things like that," he says, "my kids love them now." Celebrated Boston chef Barbara Lynch, says of her daughter, Marchesa, "She's slowly getting a palate. She still doesn't like pepper, it's too strong for her, so anything spicy she doesn't like and she loves bitter foods."

Children can begin to taste the subtleties and complexities of food, but they still prefer certain foods based on the diet they have been exposed to. "Her own palate, I don't know," says Lynch. "She's eating what we're eating. If I was cooking a lot of Indian food and Indian spices, she'd be eating that, but I don't do that often." Eric Bromberg, chef and cofounder of Blue Ribbon restaurants in New York, talks about a time before he had his own children and being with his sushi restaurant partner, Toshi: "His kids were five and seven years old and were eating raw squid and raw tuna. . . . At first it was just really startling, like,

> "If they see you enjoying something, they want to know what it is."
>
> —Floyd Cardoz, New York City chef

wow! That's unbelievable! And then we were thinking, well, that's what their dad gives them and that's how they learn what food is."

Five is a fun age also because, for the first time, I can just ask Cody outright something like, "Do you want some Brie cheese on your bread?" and there's a good chance he will give a straight—and even affirmative—answer without there being more complicated issues involved. It goes over better if it's something we can share. At this age, finally, he's more open, just thinks it over, and lets me know what he wants. His mannerisms and speaking patterns at five are almost like an adult's in many ways—he's descriptive and articulate.

Some children remain hesitant about trying foods and eating vegetables. Chef Cathal Armstrong, of Alexandria, Virginia, says, "From what I understand, kids don't taste food the same way we do, so if they find something offensive today, a month from now they may not. . . . Once you find things that they like, you build on it from there. If they won't eat a vegetable, try it again at a later date. Eventually they will come around to it as their palates grow and develop."

Cardoz says he tries foods repeatedly, but "I'll put it [on their plate] after they've forgotten about it."

It's important to note that chefs don't hide vegetables as purees in other foods for their children. "It's best for kids to understand food in its natural form and recognize it for what it is and eat it because they enjoy eating it and not try to trick them and play games with it," says Armstrong.

Chef and award-winning cookbook author Peter Berley says kids will just turn up their noses at

something and won't want to eat it, but there are vegetables that can be palatable for children, like broccoli and green beans because they are not bitter. "Broccoli stems especially have a sweetness to them because there is a carbohydrate in there. Peel the stalks and steam them or blanch them along with the florets. Children also love cooked onions because they are sweet." He acknowledges that children, being children, have food preferences. He lists other foods kids love: "any grain because grains are loaded with carbohydrates; anything milky; tofu, which is bland; sour tastes—they love pickles! They love lemon on things, salty tastes and sweet tastes. . . . Later they start to get into spicier foods and the bitter greens." He says you have to wait until they are ready for bitter flavors. "You can't force it on them." When his daughters were six or seven years old, "they started eating bitter greens like crazy. They ate lots of vegetables, including kale, collard greens, mustard greens, broccoli, and cauliflower."

Linton Hopkins's children also enjoy vegetables. He says, "We buy organic vegetables. . . . We try to buy what looks great and alive at the grocery store, and then with the kids I'll go and visit the farms. . . . They know the farmers, so they're proud to say, 'Hey, that kale is from Joe and Judith!' and there's a pride in eating it. . . . You have to buy the best ingredients and treat them simply, and then season correctly, not overcook vegetables. You cook them until they're just done so they're still bright green and alive and there's a little 'toothsomeness' to them. I think people don't know what to do with raw vegetables. I think

"We'll introduce aspects of the salad, like tomatoes. We'll get her to eat that. Then we'll try a piece of onion, and she'll try that. Gradually you just build the whole thing into a salad over a period of time."

—Cathal Armstrong, chef and co-owner of Restaurant Eve; Eamonn's, a Dublin Chipper; and The Majestic in Alexandria, Virginia

there's a real inability to approach them simply, like sautéing fennel in olive oil until it's just cooked the right way and then adding fresh lemon and parsley. It is something my kids will eat and love, but it's fresh and cooked right."

Lynch also prepares vegetables simply for Marchesa, who at six still likes to separate her foods. "If it's tomatoes, no basil on them. Maybe when she's seven she'll have basil on them."

Paul Virant, executive chef at Vie restaurant in Chicago, says that frozen vegetables are just as nutritious as fresh vegetables. Frozen broccoli, for example, is frozen one day off the farm, whereas some supermarkets have produce that, while fresh, has been off the farm for weeks. Vegetables lose their nutrients the longer they sit in trucks and on shelves.

For more challenging vegetables, like okra, Cardoz makes soup. He says his kids would never eat okra because "okra is a very hard thing to like. They tried it once and said, 'We don't like it,' and that's fine. So I made gumbo. I put the okra in there, and they ate it. They loved it. So much so, that now my eldest son loves okra."

Cooking at Home

The way chefs cook at home for their families varies. Berley cooked foods that his family found comforting and familiar—simple, healthy staples that were easy to prepare. He says kids aren't bothered by eating the same foods repeatedly because "they love repetition. . . . They don't like variety because it's scary. It's new, it's different. They think, 'Will I like this thing?' When they see the same thing that they like, it's comforting.

It's like reading children a story; they want to hear the same story every night. They know every word of the story, but they like to hear it."

But Lynch brings up an important point when she says, "If you're not cooking all the time and you're just making the basics . . . you get into a rut or a routine. So I kind of think it's important, on the weekends, just to experiment a little bit, get the kids involved."

"Kids are still kids and it has to be a pleasant experience," says Armstrong. "It's okay to battle from time to time. Once a month I'll cook something that they are not familiar with and they haven't tried before, and it's going to be a little bit of a challenge with them. For the most part I cook things I know they want to eat and maintain the dining experience as a pleasant experience." Of course chefs have a larger repertoire than most of us, and the variety of foods their children are familiar with and enjoy are also much greater than most families' handful of staple recipes.

I find Cody gets overwhelmed if we are constantly trying out too many new recipes, especially if they are exotic foods or foods that are completely out of his comfort zone. If he has had a week of eating dishes he likes, trying something new is a welcome and fun adventure.

Virant says, "One of the things that's interesting is when I cook at home it's never the same. I think that there's something good about that, and there's

"If kids have a bad experience with food, they are not going to eat it. My son, for the longest time, wouldn't eat shrimp because my mom made it once with extra salt. I had to convince him to just *try* a piece of shrimp, that it was not salty. And when he finally got over the fear, he started eating it again."

—Floyd Cardoz, New York City chef

something bad about that. I think that it's important for kids to have memories of certain foods. . . . My mom would make chicken and dumplings and pot roast—I can still taste those dishes, and they were always the same. I think there's something to be said for creating food memories." For him, cooking at home means improvising with ingredients on hand, and even if his children really like the meal, he can't necessarily re-create it. His wife is the one who uses recipes, so her dishes turn out the same way each time she makes them.

Food Associations

This age can be tricky because kids can make strong memorable associations with food. It's one thing to try to convince a toddler to try something; it's another thing altogether to convince a strong-willed six- or seven-year-old. Children can get ideas about food and develop dislikes from their friends or even from characters in movies and on television. I have a friend whose daughter suddenly refused to eat tomatoes, saying only, "I hate tom-ah-toes" in a pretend English accent by way of explanation. Eventually my friend discovered her daughter was modeling the behavior of a TV character who says that very thing in just that way.

I make Lynch's Japanese Pancakes (see page 154) a lot because it's a fun, fast dinner we all like. Once, however, I was trying out a different batter and a different method, using forms that shaped the pancakes into perfect circles. I didn't use the forms correctly, though. I put too much batter in, and the resulting pancakes were thick and a bit mushy in the

middle. The new batter wasn't great either. Usually I would say something like, "Well, it's not as good, but try it with sauce." We'd find a way to salvage it, because that's the meal I had prepared and I don't like throwing away food. But at this age, kids remember negative food experiences like that, and after one bad batch of pancakes, Cody doesn't want them at all anymore. I have a hard time convincing him that although something we tried one time wasn't good, it is good this time.

Fortunately, making memories with food goes the other way, too. Cardoz says cooking with kids, making foods they enjoy, like homemade macaroni and cheese, creates positive food associations.

Teaching Children the Culture of Food

At this age children are conversational, and it's likely that they are spending most of the day at school and then with friends. Eating meals together takes on more significance and becomes family time. "When all four of us are home together, it's an important time," says Hopkins, "and we sit down and talk and we share. I really believe in the etiquette of sitting down and having a meal together. Even if it's just twenty minutes." Armstrong believes in the importance of "being able to sit around the table and discuss social issues and current affairs, homework, school friends, and books." He calls it "the social notion of food," where eating a meal together is a pastime.

Executive chef at San Francisco's Incanto restaurant Chris Cosentino says, "My mother was an amazing single mom, and my grandparents were very close to us. We spent every Sunday sitting down as a family, sitting there having supper, and that's a big deal. I think that's part of our culture that's missing these days. That meal period with three generations sitting together is going away, and I think that's a sad part of our generation, missing out on that. We do Sundays at my house now, spending that time is really, really key. Without that, things backfire—you don't have that social family time."

Inspire Kids to Eat—with Enthusiasm!

"You put food on the table, they're gonna find their way," says Hopkins. But it is hard to watch your child refuse food, and it's hard to have to throw away uneaten food. Not every meal at this age will go well, and my husband likes to quote a funny scene in a *Desperate Housewives* episode where the culinarily high-minded Bree brings out a sumptuous

BASIC FIXES FOR COOKING MISTAKES

Good-tasting food is balanced, meaning not too sweet, salty, bitter, or sour. It is possible to fix dishes with simple additions to make them taste better. Add "fix ingredients" in small amounts, then taste and keep adjusting, if necessary.

•• Too salty: **Add a bit of sugar and/or some lemon juice or vinegar (balsamic vinegar will add both at the same time).**

•• Too sweet: **Add salt and vinegar or lemon juice. You can also add a bit of butter or cream if appropriate.**

•• Too sour: **Add a bit of salt and sugar.**

•• Too rich: **Add a bit of vinegar, lemon juice, wine, or even tomatoes.**

•• Too spicy: **Add something sweet like sugar, honey, or maple syrup, or something creamy, like yogurt or sour cream, to make spicy food taste less spicy.**

•• Too gamey: **Add or serve with something sweet, like roasted apple or roasted squash.**

Overcooked foods are inevitable from time to time in busy households where it's hard to concentrate on cooking times. And they are trickier to rescue. Meat that is overcooked won't ever become tender or succulent, but it can be made palatable. You can use overcooked meat in a soup in small pieces, or try resting very thin slices in a sauce before serving. Another option is to make a filling for something like tacos— you can add lots of fresh vegetables to contribute moisture. Whip together some chicken salad with your overcooked chicken. Puree your overcooked vegetables for a side dish or cream soup by adding some herbs and spices, cream, and/or butter. Alternatively, they can be added to a potpie or quiche.

BARBARA LYNCH is regarded as one of the country's best chefs. Her culinary empire in the Boston area includes 9 Park, named Best New Restaurant by *Food & Wine* magazine the year it opened, and she has a handful of other restaurants, a wine bar, a drink shop, a butcher shop, a modern diner, a catering company, and a cooking demonstration kitchen called Stir. She is a 2003 James Beard Award winner as Best Chef Northeast and was awarded *Food & Wine*'s 10 Best New Chefs Award. In 2009, Lynch was honored to receive the Crittenton Women's Union's Amelia Earhart Award. Past recipients include Doris Kearns Goodwin and Julia Child. Lynch's first cookbook, *Stir: Mixing It Up in the Italian Tradition,* received a prestigious Gourmand award for Best Chef Cookbook for the United States. She has a daughter, Marchesa. Lynch says, "I'm always cooking. I'm either at home cooking or we're at a gathering and I'm cooking. I make Marchesa try everything. . . . She eats oysters, shrimp cocktail, artichokes, and fried calamari. When she's with me in the different restaurants, with another friend, she's much more adventurous."

Chef Barbara Lynch : Deborah Jones

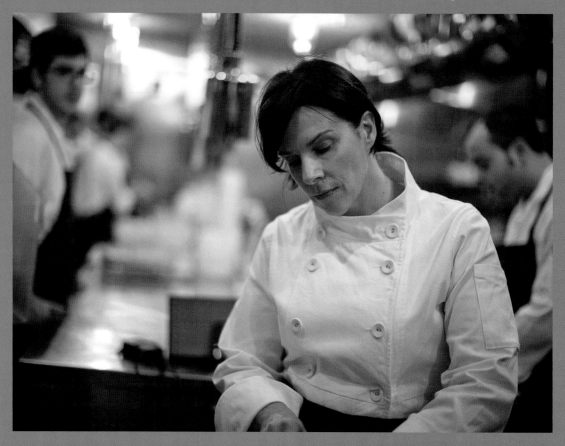

"gourmet" meal she's prepared to her family, waiting hungry at the dinner table. Andrew, her teenage son, says, "Can't we just have a hamburger and get it over with?"

Chefs inspire their own kids to eat in lots of different ways. Virant brings his family and friends to his restaurant on nights when it is closed, to cook then eat together. Lynch makes it fun for her and Marchesa to cook together and says "I got her to eat quail one night. I said, 'Look at this, this is such good chicken, this is chicken for little kids, look you can eat the whole thigh and the drumsticks.' "

Healthy Eating and Teaching Kids about Foods That Are Good for Them

Food plays a central role in children's healthy development. At this age children need to be taught not just about what healthy food is but also about not eating too many sugary foods, which profoundly impact their mood and their ability to concentrate. Kids love sugary foods.

"Taking as much sugar as possible out of the diet is important because kids already get enough sugar from other sources," says Armstrong. He is careful about the foods he buys for his household and says one of the biggest challenges as a parent is the eating habits children form outside the home. "School meals consist of sugar mixed with sugar seasoned with sugar," he says.

Lynch prefers giving her daughter, Marchesa, honey. "I love honey. I'd rather have her eat honey than mounds of sugar," she says. Sally Kravich, a natural health expert, adds that honey is actually very healthy for the body. She also suggests using a bit of date sugar or molasses or even stevia, an alternative plant-derived sweetener, instead of white sugar.

Bromberg tries to avoid serving sweet breakfasts and instead serves eggs or toast and every now and again bacon. He says, "I think there's an enormous impact to how my kids act and deal with the day based on what they're eating and how they're energized—and how they process the energy."

"It's important to get off sugar because that will create more moodiness," says Kravich. "What they all need are those fatty acids, like fish oil, that help balance hormones and calm the brain. Sugar is anti-hormone. Calcium is literally and figuratively your body's support—it emotionally supports, it keeps calmness, and it helps build bones. Dairy and fish are both good sources of calcium; almonds have calcium, too. The vegetable with the highest amount of calcium is bok choy. It is important to feed children at this age foods high in calcium, but because we can't get enough from our food, it's a good idea to also give them calcium supplements. Kids who are more hyperactive or have ADD burn calcium at a faster clip and need more calcium than the average child. The energy needs to be redirected, too, in physical activities like karate or gymnastics."

I teach Cody about the foods we're eating. I tell him proteins like beans and meats make him grow strong; vegetables, especially the green ones, make him feel good and keep him healthy; and carbohydrates like pasta and bread give him energy for running around.

ERIC BROMBERG and his twin brother, **BRUCE,** have built a small empire in New York's restaurant scene with their casual and eclectic Blue Ribbon restaurants, which include a sushi bar, a bakery, and a popular cafe serving American fare. Their restaurants are neighborhood favorites and have won a slew of awards. Bromberg is coauthor of *Bromberg Bros. Blue Ribbon Cookbook*. He is the father of three children: Leah, Jason, and Brett. "I love everything about food and cultures, and I'm more interested in food from different places than anything," he says. Of his children's eating, he says, "They'll taste anything, some things they'll spit out and say, 'that was disgusting,' but they'll try just about anything." Jason, Bromberg's son, says, "Sometimes the best thing is the thing that looks horrible. I remember my first time trying asparagus, I'm, like, 'Ew, I don't wanna try that!' and then, when I tried it, I found out that it was really good!" Bromberg adds, "Jason had seaweed soup and thought it was going to be gross, and he didn't try it the first time at all. And then the second time, he tried it and decided it was pretty cool. We order anything; I am as adventurous as I can be."

Eric Bromberg and son Jason at Blue Ribbon : MARY ANN MARINO

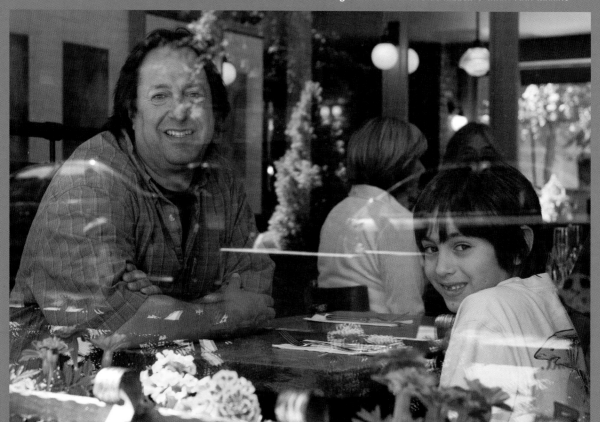

Bromberg says his children "actually often ask, 'What's good for me?' and 'What's not good for me?' . . . And we do our best to suggest that everything is essentially good for you, it's just a question of quantity. So sugar isn't bad for you, but too much sugar is bad for you. Salt's not bad for you, too much salt is bad for you. Fat isn't bad for you, it's too much of it that is." Jason, Bromberg's son, says he went through a phase in which he wanted to have strawberry milk for all his meals. "I'd never really eat anything, I'd have strawberry milk and say, 'I'm full!'" says Jason. It was a learning experience says Bromberg. "We talked about it and he chose that—that's what he wanted to eat, and we did that for a while." But then Jason got a cavity. "We just told him if he kept drinking strawberry milk, then he was going to get more cavities. . . . Something happened and he kind of learned it. It just seems to me to be a much more successful way of teaching. . . . So, I take that approach with most things." Jason, at the end of the story, proudly says, "I don't drink any type of flavored milk except for plain, just plain milk."

Children at this age can learn about the importance of reading labels at the grocery store and making decisions about what to eat and not eat, what's fun and what looks fun but isn't wholesome or healthy food.

"I'm a firm anti–high fructose corn syrup guy," says Cardoz. "I look at all my labels. We have only organic unsweetened ketchup at home, there's no Heinz ketchup. My kids are allowed to have a soda only once a week at home. . . . When their friends come over, it becomes an issue, and it gets a little hard. Instead, at home my kids drink fresh orange

"I know some parents who don't allow their kids to have any candy and with some success. They don't allow it in any form. But I think it's pretty complicated, especially when a kid isn't with you and candy is available. I think it just creates a really weird relationship. So we let our kids have, pretty much, what they like to eat, and I think it encourages them to eat other things that they don't know whether they're going to like. And they'll always, especially Jason, try anything."

—Eric Bromberg, chef and cofounder of New York City's Blue Ribbon restaurants

juice—we squeeze it ourselves. They eat fruit . . . there's always fruit in the home. And there are always vegetables. There're going to be times when they fail, and you have to let them, in moderation. You've got to help them make right choices."

Five-year-olds can be stubborn about eating, Kravich says, and sometimes a psychological way of talking works. She tells a story about a five-year-old girl she was working with. Like many young children, she had a preference for sugary breakfast cereals, and her mother had a hard time convincing her to eat things like oatmeal. "I talked to the little girl about a lot of different things, but the first thing I said was, 'Are you the mommy or is she the mommy?' She said, 'She's the mommy, silly.' So I said, 'Mommies need to

> "We're focused on food tasting good and on having the right amount of food that makes you feel comfortable and not feel sick after eating and simplifying meals at home, so there's not a conflict or a battle."
>
> —Eric Bromberg, chef and co-owner of New York City's Blue Ribbon restaurants

show you what to do so *you* can grow up to be a good mommy.'" Kravich adds that parents are sometimes too permissive with their kids, allowing their kids to determine the foods they eat without any real regulation or guidance or even allowing them to eat too many snack foods in lieu of meals for example.

Cardoz, like most chefs, stays away from fast food. His son, Peter, was seeing lots of McDonald's advertising on children's programs and wanted to eat there all the time. "We didn't cut it off totally," Cardoz says. "I felt Peter would not be too happy, and it was the right way to go about it. We cut it down tremendously. We would give it to them occasionally but not often . . . these things are not taught to kids. I feel it's up to the parent to make sure and teach what is acceptable and what is not." Cardoz doesn't buy many processed foods either and says, "Sometimes my son wants to have one of those breakfast things, Pop-tarts, that you put in the toaster oven. And we let him have that because all the kids in school are having that. We don't ban it totally. Occasionally the kids are allowed to have them."

Armstrong says what's important for him is to "maintain that they eat a balanced diet: some proteins, some carbohydrates, some vitamins, some minerals." Lynch calls herself a healthy eater, "so it's important that whatever I'm feeding myself and my husband, we feed Marchesa the same. It's important because we want to eat together." When Berley's children were young, "We tried to emphasize home-cooked food. We never told them what to eat when they weren't at home with us, so there was nothing for them to rebel against. Not wanting to stigmatize them or make them feel like there were taboos on food . . . when they were on their own they ate whatever they wanted." Armstrong points out that children at this age have a tendency to rebel against their parents, "so I've really tried not to be overly aggressive with any information I'm giving them, but just to show them."

B. T. Nguyen, chef and owner of Restaurant BT in Tampa, believes it was important to carefully nurture and develop her children's palates through their infancy and younger years because it would make them choose to eat good, healthy foods when they began to make their own decisions about eating. She says when her children were about seven or eight years old, "they wanted control over what they wanted to eat, and I gave it to them. Okay now you want to take over—go ahead. I think *you* should have that experience."

Some kids still don't eat a lot at mealtimes. "When she's full, she's full," says Lynch of her daughter, Marchesa. "She noshes all day, but it depends if she has gymnastics or lots of activities at school that day. It depends if she's going through a growth spurt, too."

PAUL VIRANT grew up in Missouri, where his grandmothers took him to the local smoke-house and farmers' market and taught him how to preserve fruit and pickle vegetables. He is the chef/owner of a restaurant just outside Chicago named Vie, which means "life" in French. He says of his restaurant, "I wanted to create an extension of my home, where people can come and enjoy good food and drink in the company of the people whom they care about. And I want them to enjoy every morsel and drop of life." His awards include being named Best New Chef 2007 by *Food & Wine* magazine. He has competed several times on the Food Network's *Iron Chef* and is the father of two boys, Zane and Lincoln.

Paul Virant and his sons, Lincoln and Zane : LINDA BERGONIA

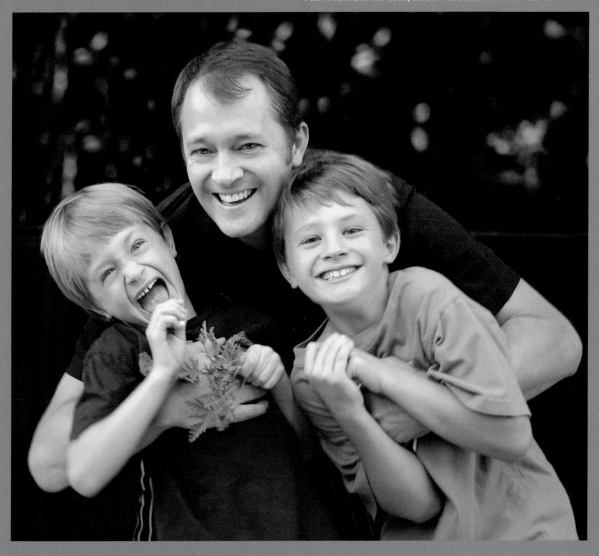

Chef Paul Virant recommends similar strategies for feeding big kids as for little ones. As children grow and develop, they take more in from, say, a visit to the farm, and they can take on more responsibility in caring for a garden. Utensils are no longer just toys; they can handle a knife to cut their own food.

- Mix it up. Serving a variety of foods is important, including a broad range of ingredients, flavors, and fine foods.

- Cook foods simply. Make a simple chicken dish and add a flavorful relish for the children to taste and the adults to enjoy.

- Be accommodating. It's important to take the kids' preferences into account when making meals.

- Teach. Exposing children to all stages of food production from seed to table is important. Take a trip to the farm or plant a small garden.

- Serve family style meals. Put food on large plates in the center of the table and let everyone take what they like.

- Get special utensils. Give kids fun forks or a special kids' knife like the Kuhn Ricon Kinderkitchen kids' knife or colorful one-piece learning chopsticks.

Table Rules

For Virant, dinner lasts about a half hour. His table rules are to sit up straight and keep your napkin on your lap, and he still has to remind his kids frequently.

"I think the most important thing for parents," says Armstrong, "is to be confident, consistent, and patient." All chefs agree that mealtimes require patience. Taking time out for dinner is important, but sometimes children need to be reminded repeatedly about things like using utensils and staying seated.

"Our biggest thing," says Hopkins, "is you can't leave the table until you've tried at least two bites of everything. But sometimes they're just not hungry; they may have a yogurt before dinner that really fills them up. So they may just eat five or seven bites and they're done."

Lots of children need help to focus on eating. Children do best when dinner is served early. They get hungry around five and want to eat. Eating snacks before dinner is common, and Lynch limits bread before meals so Marchesa eats more of the prepared foods. Bromberg says, "We have dinnertime, and when you get up from the table and you're done, that's your dinner and then you do a couple of things and you do your homework and you get ready for bed. At bedtime you don't say, 'I'm hungry, I didn't have anything for dinner.' Ninety-nine percent of the time that gets the message across that you eat what you're hungry for and that's it. It's not just a casual thing where if you feel like you're hungry at eight o'clock when it's time to go to bed you can have another dinner. That doesn't mean that we don't have late-night snacks as well sometimes . . . like an apple or a banana. We definitely make it so they don't eat before bed, 'cause that always kind of has a rough-night's-sleep effect."

If Cody is not engaged in the cooking process, but is playing by himself, and I call him to the table and just put a plate of food down in front of him, then eating is not something he will want to do. He'd rather not be interrupted, even for meatballs—his favorite. If I connect him in some way to the meal preparation, it goes better. When he's participated, he feels he has more of a say and he's included. I find if I sit with him where he's playing and talk to him for a couple of minutes before I start cooking and tell him what I'm thinking of making for dinner, he'll wander over to the kitchen himself for a bit while I'm cooking. He'll drive his toy car over and jump up on a stool to see what's in the pan. I make room for him and let him mix, pour stuff into the pot, or grate cheese if he wants to.

"We get through the point of one kid saying, 'Oh, I hate that,' when the other two like it or he liked it last week. As long as you're not really engaged [in] that part of the conversation when they're sitting at the table anyway, then eventually they settle down, they get hungry, and they'll eat what they like or what they want," says Bromberg.

Shopping with Kids

The experience of grocery shopping with kids can be challenging. They see endless aisles stacked top to bottom with colorful bags, boxes, and jars, and it seems like a free-for-all to reach for anything they want and throw it in the basket. It's very stimulating for Cody, and in every aisle he randomly grabs

"We go to the supermarket together, and that's a really positive thing. We always go through the vegetable section and the meat section and the fish section, and I ask them what this vegetable is or that vegetable is and they know almost all the vegetables."

—Eric Bromberg, chef and co-owner of New York City's Blue Ribbon restaurants

things within his reach. He is constantly asking for things that look fun or that he recognizes from being with his friends. Of course he likes all the cartoons on the cereal boxes, and he doesn't understand why we buy what we buy, and it raises a lot of questions. Sometimes we turn it around and draw large pictures of animals like panda bears and elephants to cut out and put on our more homely looking breakfast cereal boxes. We make up our own names and stories as we're eating breakfast.

Chefs have an advantage because they navigate grocery stores looking for raw ingredients like vegetables and meats, or unflavored and unprocessed ingredients like pasta or rolled oats. Preparing most of their meals from scratch simplifies shopping because they can avoid the aisles of processed foods, which are usually packaged to draw the attention of children, with designs of cartoon characters and colorful pictures. "Lunchables are a very good example of marketing to kids," says Hopkins, "and I swear even now my kids walk by and they're like 'Lunchables!'

DIANE FORLEY and **MICHAEL OTSUKA** were co-executive chefs of the critically acclaimed restaurant Verbena. Forley was named one of America's Hottest Young Chefs by the *Wine Spectator* and is the author of *Anatomy of a Dish.* Forley's influences include her parents' Egyptian, Guatemalan, and Hungarian ancestry. Otsuka has a Japanese American father and a Viennese Jewish mother. He learned to make traditional Japanese dishes with his paternal grandmother. They now have bakery in Scarsdale, New York, called Flourish Baking Company. Forley and Otsuka have lots of ethnic spices in their pantry and bring foods into the house that they love to eat. They prepare foods from scratch, and they believe food should taste good. Their two children have different eating behaviors. When Otsuka used to go fishing, his daughter, Olivia, who is a super smeller and a more discerning eater, was fascinated with the fish he brought home. She'd want to look it over and touch it, but she wouldn't eat it. But Adam, their son who eats lots of different things, loves to eat fish.

Diane Forley and Michael Otsuka with daughter Olivia and son Adam : MARY ANN MARINO

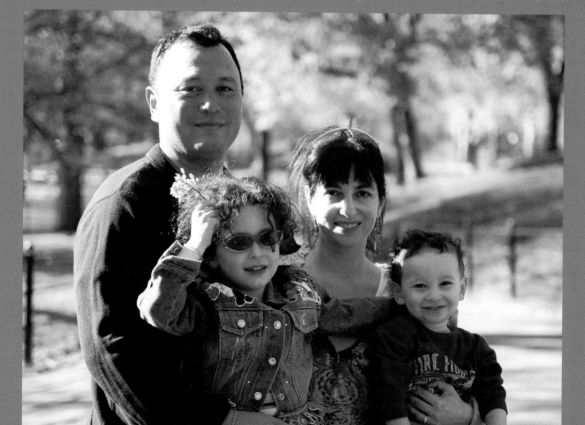

and I say, 'Are you kidding me? No way!' They're starting to fade away from asking that every time."

Hopkins teaches his children about foods when he helps them make selections at the store. "Avery made a choice. We usually get just plain applesauce, and she actually got the stuff with cinnamon, and I was fine with that as long as it was still all natural, organic applesauce with no sugar added. The big thing for us is a lot of added sugar. We put a cap on the number of grams of sugar a cereal can have per serving, and there can be no high-fructose corn syrup in anything. We really try to control things that way." And Hopkins adds, "I'm not the bad guy. The label is. So, if they see ingredients on the label that they don't know how to pronounce, we're not eating it."

Kravich says that MSG, a prevalent food additive and common flavor enhancer in fast foods and packaged and manufactured foods, can overwhelm taste buds. And it's true that kids who continually munch on BBQ potato chips have a hard time transitioning to more sophisticated and wholesome flavors.

Kravich points out that MSG oftentimes isn't listed on food ingredient lists as such and may be listed as "natural flavorings," hydrolyzed protein, or even simply as "spices."

"The first thing we hit is the vegetable section, always," Hopkins says. A good reason to start there is that it's so colorful. Kravich points out that kids are associative in their thinking, and if you take them to the vegetable section first, it becomes first in their consciousness. Also, she says, kids have a limited attention span, so if you're hitting the important things first, that's what they'll see. It satisfies Cody, who helps pick the vegetables and fruits that fill the basket. "Children want to participate in the process," says Hopkins, "and letting them helps them learn in little steps . . . the whole culture of going through a grocery store where kids are saying, 'I want.' You know, it's not just long lists of 'I want,' and you get everything you want down every aisle."

Cardoz allows his children to select things they want, and then they go home and cook them together.

chicken with lemon, artichokes, and parsley

{ JENNIFER VIRANT, CHEF PAUL VIRANT'S WIFE }

SERVES 4

This is a shockingly fast dinner to cook and so surprisingly good it's become part of our regular repertoire. It's equally tasty with either boneless chicken breasts or bone-in, skin-on breasts—the skin is perfectly cooked and the meat tender and full of flavor. For bone-in, simply increase the cooking time by 5 minutes.

3 skinless, boneless chicken breasts

Salt and pepper

2 tablespoons butter

1 14-ounce can artichoke hearts (packed in water), drained and quartered

¾ cup chopped, loosely packed Italian parsley

½ lemon, juiced

1. Pound breasts a bit so they are no more than 1-inch thick and season with salt and pepper on both sides. If using bone-in, rub salt and pepper on the skin on bottom sides.

2. Preheat a large saucepan to medium heat and, when hot, add butter.

3. Add chicken to the pan to brown smooth-side down or skin-side down if using bone-in. Cover with a lid, and cook for about 5 minutes, or an extra 3 minutes longer for bone-in.

4. Flip chicken over, add artichoke hearts, and cover again to cook for another 3 minutes, or an extra 5 minutes for bone-in; then add the parsley and lemon juice. Cook uncovered for 1 minute more and serve.

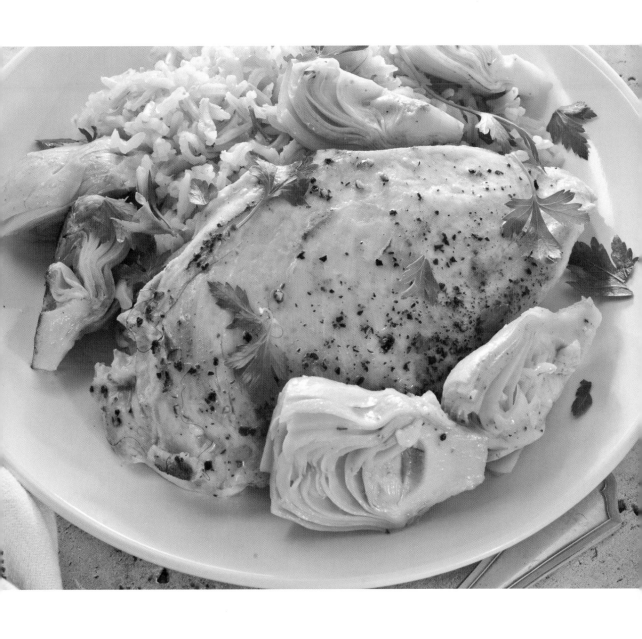

braised chicken with farro, tuscan kale, tomatoes, and parmigiana reggiano

{ PAUL VIRANT }

SERVES 4

This is made in one pot—a true masterpiece dish, both beautiful to serve and deeply satisfying to eat for a nice stay-at-home dinner. The chicken is succulent, and the skin gets perfectly crisped. It feels like a very elegant meal, even though it is quite simple to make.

Note: Farro is a healthy whole grain that can be found at Whole Foods or similar markets. It has a hearty, rustic, nutty flavor and is served like rice.

4 chicken leg and thigh quarters

Salt and pepper

¼ cup plus 2 tablespoons extra-virgin olive oil

1 sweet onion, sliced

7 cloves garlic, sliced

2 teaspoons sweet smoked paprika

¾ cup farro

1 tablespoon chopped thyme

1 cup Italian white wine (Pinot Grigio)

¼ pound Tuscan kale, stems removed, leaves chopped small

1 cup diced tomatoes

3 cups chicken stock

2 tablespoons chopped Italian parsley

Parmigiana Reggiano

1. Season legs and thighs with salt and pepper. Over medium-high heat brown the chicken in ¼ cup olive oil in a Dutch oven, about 5 minutes per side. Remove chicken to a plate. Add onions, garlic, and paprika to the Dutch oven and cook a few minutes.

2. Preheat oven to 350°F.

3. Add farro and thyme, cook another minute. Add white wine; bring to a boil and cook until the liquid has reduced and its flavor has concentrated. Add kale and tomatoes, cover, and cook for 5 minutes.

4. Place chicken back in the pot, add chicken stock, bring to a boil, and place in the oven. Cook uncovered for 45 minutes in the oven, until the farro is done and most of the liquid has evaporated.

5. Remove from oven and add parsley and remaining 2 tablespoons of olive oil; season with salt and pepper.

6. Arrange farro and Tuscan kale on a serving platter, place chicken on top. Garnish with a generous amount of grated Parmigiana Reggiano, and serve.

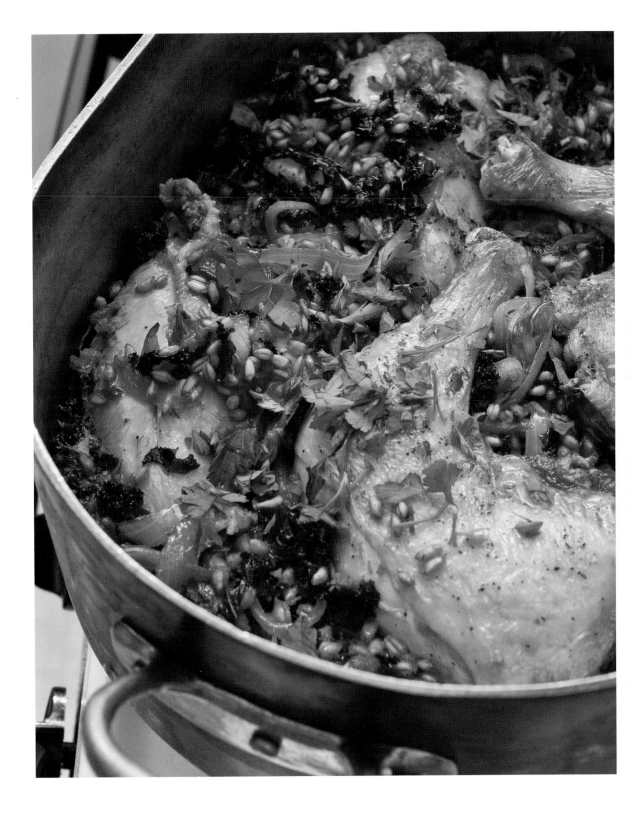

chocolate fillet of prime beef

{ JIMMY SCHMIDT }

SERVES 4

Chef Jimmy Schmidt uses certified Angus beef, which is a premium meat that boasts superior flavor and tenderness. He suggests a simple melted chocolate sauce.

For adults, try sautéing half an onion and some garlic in butter, then adding half a cup each white wine and water, reducing, then adding the chocolate and seasoning with salt and pepper.

Steaks:

1½ teaspoons natural cocoa powder

½ teaspoon sea salt

1½ teaspoons sugar

4 fillets of prime tenderloin of beef, about 4 ounces each

1 teaspoon safflower oil

Glaze:

4 ounces milk chocolate, melted

Chocolate milk as necessary for consistency

1. Preheat broiler on the lower setting, about 460°F.

2. Mix the cocoa powder, salt, and sugar together in a bowl. Rub the steaks with safflower oil and then roll the steaks in the spices to coat all surfaces lightly. Tap to remove any excess.

3. To make the glaze, melt chocolate in a small pan over very low heat. When melted add enough chocolate milk to make it into a sauce.

4. Place the steaks in an ovenproof pan and put under the broiler. Cook until seared but not heavily browned, about 6 minutes. Turn over and continue to cook, approximately 4 minutes for medium rare, depending on the heat of your broiler and thickness of your steak. Remove the steaks from the oven, brush with glaze, and let rest for a couple of minutes.

5. After the steaks have rested, cut into easy-to-eat slices and arrange in a fan on a serving plate; drizzle the remaining sauce over them.

kaffir lime leaf shrimp

{ B. T. NGUYEN }

SERVES 4

Kaffir lime leaves are incredibly fragrant, and the use of them removes any fishy smell from the shrimp. I like making this with kid-size shrimp. Serve these shrimp with rice. This recipe calls for using sugar cane sticks as skewers. It's delicious to chew a bit on the skewer, and the heated sugar cane releases a burst of sweet juice, says Nguyen. We get them at the local farmers' market, where they sell fresh sugar cane juice, but it can be found canned too. Sugar cane is loaded with essential nutrients and has many health benefits. While eating refined white sugar zaps energy, sugar cane boosts energy and is actually healthy to eat. You can also use bamboo skewers.

6 fresh whole Kaffir lime leaves
1 tablespoon finely chopped garlic
1 teaspoon palm sugar
1 teaspoon pepper
1 tablespoon roasted sesame seeds
2 tablespoons pure sesame oil
2 tablespoons fish sauce
20 shrimp, peeled and deveined
4 7-inch lengths sugar cane sticks or bamboo skewers

1. Mix Kaffir lime leaves, garlic, palm sugar, pepper, sesame seeds, sesame oil, and fish sauce in a bowl; set aside.

2. Skewer 5 shrimp onto each sugar cane stick; brush shrimp skewers with Kaffir lime mixture and refrigerate for 2 to 3 hours.

3. Grill for 3 minutes on each side. (Do not overcook shrimp, or they will get chewy.) Serve with a vegetable of your choice.

sweet ginger baked tofu

{ PETER BERLEY }

SERVES 4

Cody likes this flavorful tofu a lot. We make a bunch to keep around to put in salads, have for lunch, or snack on after we've been running around. This can be served simply as an accompaniment with cold soba noodles or cut up and simmered in miso soup. If your kids are resistant to trying something new, like tofu, try to engage them in a guessing game about the ingredients. What do they taste—ginger? Honey? Sesame?

1 pound extra-firm tofu
¼ cup soy sauce
¼ cup rice vinegar
¼ cup apple cider or apple juice
2 tablespoons sesame oil or olive oil
2 tablespoons honey
1 small clove garlic, minced
1½ tablespoons minced fresh ginger

1. Preheat oven to 375°F.

2. Slice tofu ½-inch thick. Lay the tofu between two clean cotton dishtowels. Put a plate on top and a weight on the plate (a couple of cans of beans or tomatoes will do). Set aside for 15 minutes.

3. Whisk the remaining ingredients together in a bowl.

4. Lay the tofu snug together in a single layer in a rimmed baking pan. Pour on the marinade and bake on the middle shelf of the oven for 30 minutes or until the tofu is well browned and the marinade has been absorbed.

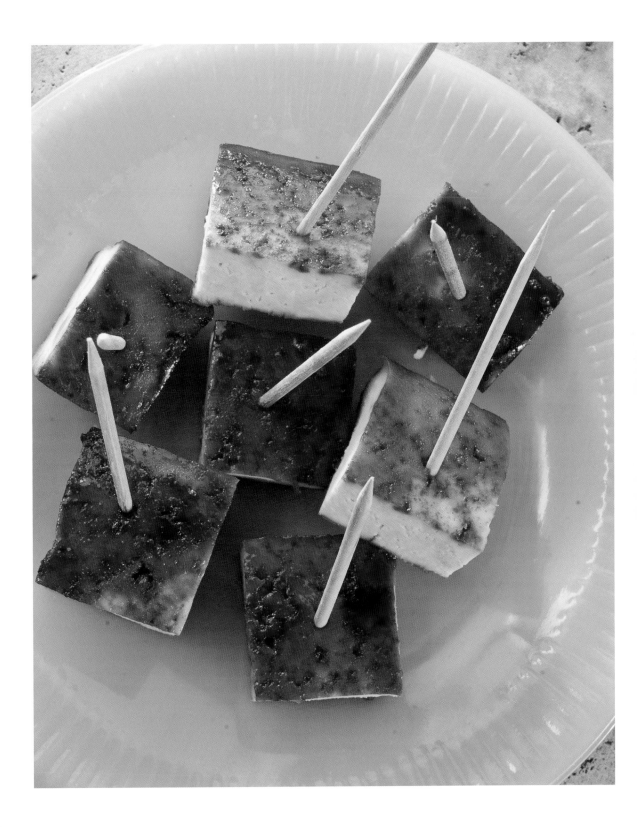

broccoli with olive oil and sea salt

{ BARBARA LYNCH }

SERVES 4

This is how Chef Barbara Lynch makes broccoli for her daughter, Marchesa. Adding good-quality olive oil and specialty salt to the vegetables makes them especially delicious. It's also a good basic preparation for other vegetables like carrots, cauliflower, and green beans. You can quickly cook a small handful of vegetables this way for an easy kid-size vegetable snack or to put in a lunchbox. Vegetables can be steamed if you have a steamer or quickly blanched in boiling water. The trick to the recipe is to use good ingredients and to cook the vegetables just right so they are still bright in color and either just cooked through or with a bit of crunch still in them, depending on your preference. Young children will enjoy drizzling the olive oil and sprinkling the sea salt. It may help get them to take that first bite.

2 heads broccoli, chopped into small florets, stems peeled and chopped
2 tablespoons best-quality extra-virgin olive oil
Good-quality sea salt

1. Steam the broccoli until just cooked through and remove to a serving plate.

2. Drizzle the olive oil over and sprinkle with sea salt.

Note: Traditional *fleur de sel* is a type of hand-harvested sea salt from France that imparts a flavor much better than that of regular table salt. Specialty salts have different shapes and have a bit of a welcome and surprising crunch. Fleur de sel has a higher mineral content than table salt and smells like the sea. It dissolves quicker than regular salt and is sprinkled on food just before serving. Try some on chocolate ice cream!

broccoli and cheese curds

{ PAUL VIRANT }

Cody liked both the cheese and the broccoli but started to separate them, saying that he liked them apart. It sparked a conversation about the way things go together and that sometimes things taste better together. We talked about BLTs being tastier because the flavor of the bacon mixes in with all the other flavors in the sandwich, like the juicy tomato and crispy lettuce. I asked him to take a mixed bite and tell me what he thought. He agreed that the cheese was good together with the broccoli.

1 tablespoon butter
½ pound broccoli (fresh or frozen), cut into florets
    and stems chopped
Salt and pepper
¼ pound cheese curds (preferably from Wisconsin)

1. Preheat oven to 400°F.

2. Heat the butter in a 10-inch skillet (preferably cast-iron) and add frozen or fresh broccoli.

3. Cook on medium-high heat until the frozen broccoli is warmed and any water evaporates. If using fresh broccoli, cook for about 3 minutes, add 1 tablespoon of water, and cover to steam for 3 to 5 minutes, until the broccoli is tender.

4. Season with salt and pepper, sprinkle curds on top, and bake for 10 minutes. Serve.

Notes: Fresh cheese curds have a mild, slightly milky flavor and a characteristic "squeak" when eaten. Unfortunately, cheese curds rapidly lose their freshness, and they should be eaten very quickly.

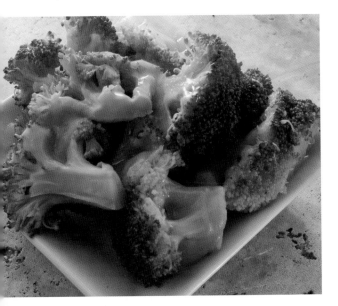

winter gratin of potato, onion, and cabbage

{ PETER BERLEY }

SERVES 4

We like serving this with sausage. It's not rich or fancy—it makes a great casual meal. The potatoes get tender and a bit sweet from the onions, and the cabbage is a bit tart. I usually don't go for bread crumbs, but these I find myself picking off first to eat, just like Cody.

4 slices sourdough bread, cut into small cubes
¼ cup extra-virgin olive oil, divided
1½ teaspoons unsalted butter
1 cup thinly sliced onion (about 1 large onion)
2 garlic cloves, finely chopped
1½ teaspoons caraway seeds
Pinch red pepper flakes
Sea salt or kosher salt
1 pound potatoes, peeled and thinly sliced crosswise
Freshly ground black pepper
¼ small head green cabbage, halved, cored, and
   sliced crosswise ⅓-inch thick (about 3 cups)
½ lemon, juiced
½ cup vegetable or chicken stock or water
¼ cup finely grated Parmesan cheese (about 2 ounces)
¼ cup coarsely grated Gruyère cheese (about 2
   ounces)

1. Set a rack in the middle of the oven and preheat to 200°F. Spread the sourdough cubes out on a baking tray and bake for 10 minutes or until dry, tossing halfway through. Remove from the oven and let cool. Crush with your hands to break up into crumbs.

2. Turn oven up to 400°F.

3. Warm 1½ teaspoons of the olive oil and the butter in a small straight-sided ovenproof skillet, preferably cast-iron. Add the onion and cook, stirring occasionally, until lightly browned, 5 to 7 minutes. Add the garlic, caraway seeds, red pepper flakes, and pinch of salt, and cook, stirring, for 1 minute. Transfer the mixture to a bowl.

4. In another large bowl, toss the potatoes with 1 tablespoon of the olive oil, and season with ½ teaspoon of salt and a generous grinding of pepper. In a third bowl, toss the cabbage with 1½ teaspoons of olive oil, lemon juice, and a pinch of salt.

5. Layer half the potatoes in the skillet. Layer in half the cabbage, then half the onion. Repeat, finishing with the onion. Pour in the stock or water.

6. In a bowl, toss the bread crumbs with the remaining olive oil and both cheeses, and season with salt and pepper.

7. Spread the bread crumb mixture over the vegetables. Place the pan over medium heat and bring the liquid to a simmer.

8. Cover and transfer to the oven and bake for 35 minutes. Remove the cover and continue to bake until the vegetables offer no resistance when pierced with a fork and the topping is crisp and golden, about another 5 minutes. Let the gratin rest for 5 to 10 minutes before serving.

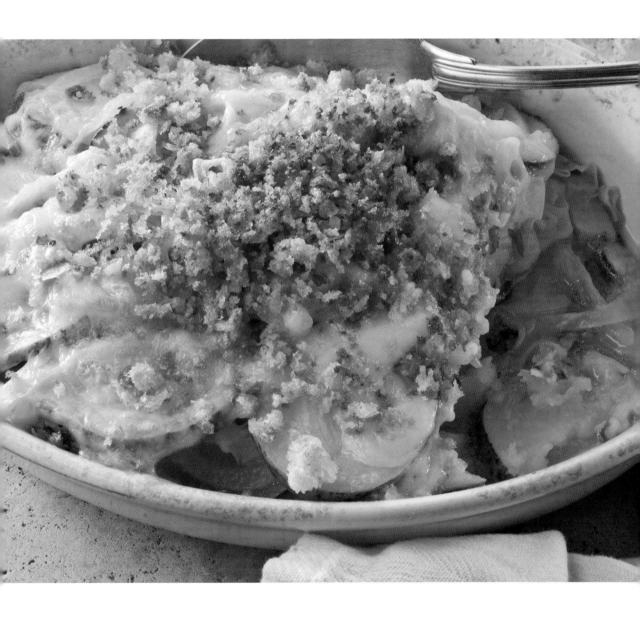

spicy tomato soup with crispy grilled cheese

{ BARBARA LYNCH }

SERVES 6

This is a delicious early weekday dinner or rainy-day lunch—the grilled cheese sandwiches are great for scooping up bites of soup. These sandwiches are a bit more work, but they are so delicious they are worth it! If you like your sandwiches extra crispy, cook them a bit longer.

Soup:

2 tablespoons extra-virgin olive oil

1 small onion, sliced

1 pinch crushed red pepper flakes (up to ½ teaspoon more if you want it spicy, as I do)

2 28-ounce cans plum tomatoes

1½ cups water

¼ cup fresh basil leaves

Kosher salt and freshly ground black pepper

Grilled Cheese:

Good country, French, or Italian bread

8 tablespoons (1 stick) unsalted butter, at room temperature

½ pound mozzarella cheese

1. To make the soup, heat the olive oil in a large, heavy saucepan over medium heat.

2. Add the onion and red pepper flakes and cook, stirring occasionally, until the onion is tender, about 7 minutes.

3. Add the tomatoes and water and cook, stirring occasionally, for 30 minutes.

4. Add the basil, season lightly with salt and pepper, and let cool briefly.

5. Puree the soup in a food processor, in batches if necessary, and pass through a fine-mesh strainer, pressing the solids with a ladle. (Save the pulp, if you like; though it has no place in this soup, it's great on crostini or baked eggplant.) Keep the soup on medium-low heat if you plan to serve it right away.

6. To make the grilled cheese, stick the bread in the freezer briefly; it will be easier to slice when cold and firm. With a serrated knife, cut the bread into 12 exceedingly thin slices—as thin as you can without making the bread fall apart.

7. Melt the butter in a skillet over medium heat.

8. Heat the oven to 400°F. Have ready two heavy baking sheets of the same size so that one can nestle into the other. Line one with a sheet of parchment paper.

9. Slice the cheese thinly. (How thin is not as crucial here, as the cheese melts so thoroughly that it practically disappears into the bread.)

10. Brush 6 of the bread slices with the melted butter and lay them butter-side down on the parchment-lined baking sheet. Top each with a single layer of cheese and then top with another slice of buttered bread to make sandwiches.

11. Put the sandwiches on the prepared baking sheet, leaving some space between them. Cover the sandwiches with a piece of parchment and stack the second baking sheet on top of the first; this will cook the sandwiches on both sides without the need to flip them and will also flatten them a bit.

12. Bake until the sandwiches are golden brown and crisp, 15 to 20 minutes.

13. Carefully peel away the top layer of parchment, transfer the sandwiches to a cooling rack, and serve warm or at room temperature. If there are any ragged bits of baked cheese hanging off the sandwiches, just trim them away by hand; you'll want to eat these, so go ahead.

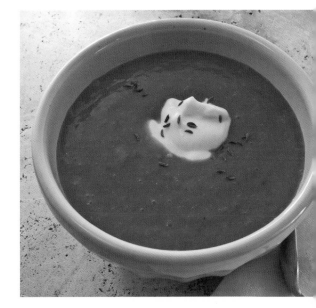

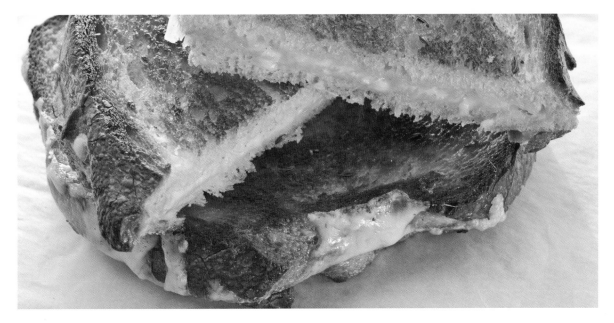

sweet red pepper linguine

{ JIMMY SCHMIDT }

This is a great dish for children who prefer very plain foods. The colorful pepper stays nicely crunchy. Sprinkle cheese on top at the table. We like serving this cold for lunch, and we use a bit less Parmesan cheese.

Sea salt

¾ pound linguine (whole wheat or high fiber preferred)

3 red bell peppers, cored and cut into fine julienne to mimic the size of the noodles

4 tablespoons unsalted butter, melted.

½ cup grated Parmesan cheese, divided

1. Bring a large pot of water to a boil. Add 1½ tablespoons salt. When the water returns to a boil, add the pasta and cook until just tender.

2. Add the red peppers to the cooking pasta for 1 minute to warm and slightly soften. Scoop out a cup of pasta water and set aside. Drain the pasta and peppers into a colander and transfer to a large bowl. Add the melted butter and half the Parmesan, tossing to coat well. Adjust the seasoning with salt as necessary and add some of the pasta water if the pasta is dry.

3. To serve, twist the noodles into a mound in the center of each plate. Sprinkle the rest of the cheese on top at the table.

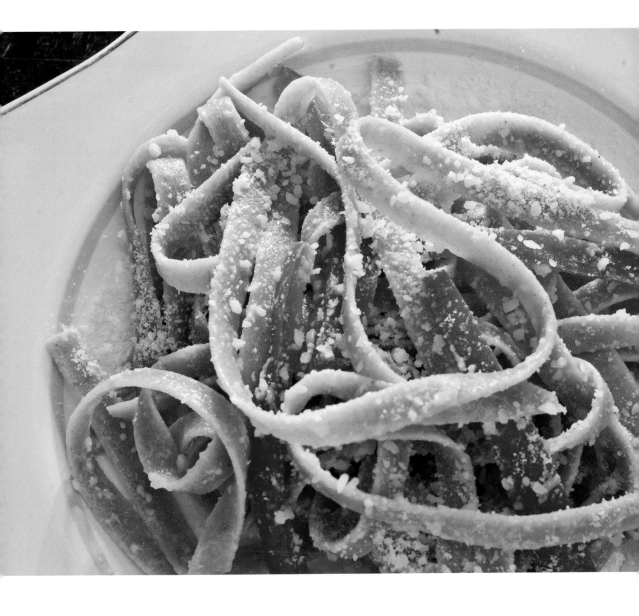

penne with bacon, peas, and lemon

{ JENNIFER VIRANT, CHEF PAUL VIRANT'S WIFE }

SERVES 4

Like all kids, Cody loves bacon, and in this dish, three of his favorite foods are brilliantly combined. Try adding mint or parsley at the end and sautéing vegetables like broccoli, asparagus, sliced brussels sprouts, or Swiss chard in the pan with the bacon fat before adding the peas.

Salt
¾ pound penne pasta
½ pound bacon, about 4 thick slices, diced
1 shallot or ½ onion, chopped
¼ cup olive oil
Juice and zest, grated, from 1 lemon
1 cup frozen peas, thawed
Salt and pepper

1. Bring a large pot of water to a boil. Add 1½ tablespoons salt. When the water returns to a boil, add the pasta and cook until just tender.

2. Meanwhile, cook the bacon in a large straight-sided skillet, and when crisp, spoon off all but approximately 1 tablespoon of the fat from the pan. Add the shallots or onions and cook until tender, about 5 minutes.

3. When the pasta is tender, before draining, scoop out a cupful of liquid and set aside. Drain the pasta.

4. Add the olive oil, lemon juice, and lemon zest to the pan with the bacon, scraping and mixing in the browned bits off the bottom of the pan.

5. Immediately add the drained pasta and the peas to the pan, stirring to combine.

6. Season with salt and pepper and add a splash of the pasta liquid if dry, and serve.

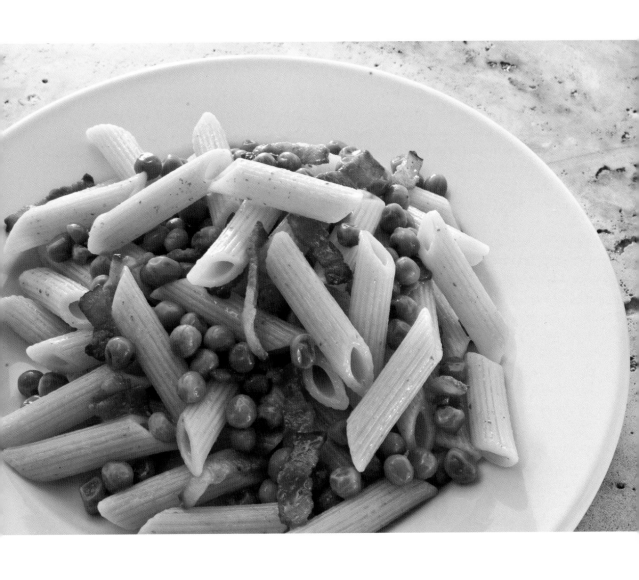

delicate ricotta gnudi

{ BARBARA LYNCH }

SERVES 4

Gnudi are the light, cloud-like cheese fillings of ravioli made to be served without their pasta sheath. Here they are prepared with a bit of flour—making them easy to work with and a great way to introduce kids to making their own pasta. They go well with lots of sauces, including a simple one of butter and sage. They need not be perfectly shaped to be tasty, so have some fun! They can be stored for several days or frozen.

½ pound ricotta, drained if very wet
¼–½ cup all-purpose flour, plus more as needed
1 large egg, lightly beaten
3 tablespoons finely grated Parmigiana Reggiano
2 teaspoons kosher salt
¼ teaspoon freshly ground white pepper

1. In a large mixing bowl, combine the ricotta, ¼ cup flour, egg, cheese, salt, and pepper. Use a wooden spoon to mix ingredients together well.

2. Lightly flour your work surface and a baking sheet for holding the shaped gnudi. With floured hands, knead the ricotta mixture briefly; it will be quite wet and sticky at this point. Dump the mixture out onto your work surface.

3. Cut off a piece of the gnudi dough and try rolling it into a ¾-inch-thick log. If you can't get it to roll, add a little more flour to the dough and try again. You want as little flour as possible to keep these together so the resulting gnudi will be light and ethereal.

4. Cut the log into 1-inch pieces and then roll into little balls. If you have a gnocchi board, hold it at a 45-degree angle over your floured baking sheet and roll each ball down the length of it to give the gnudi grooves. As the gnudi nears the end of the board, let it drop onto the baking sheet. If you don't have a gnocchi board, hold a fork, tines facing down, and roll the ball down the length of the tines. Repeat until all of the dough is rolled and cut.

5. Freeze the gnudi, about 1 hour. (Because they are so soft, they are much easier to handle frozen, so do this even if you plan to use them soon.)

6. To serve, bring a large pot of well-salted water to a gentle boil. In batches, drop the gnudi into the water and cook until they float, about 1 to 2 minutes. As each batch cooks, remove gnudi with a slotted spoon and keep them warm or transfer them directly to the sauce they are being served with.

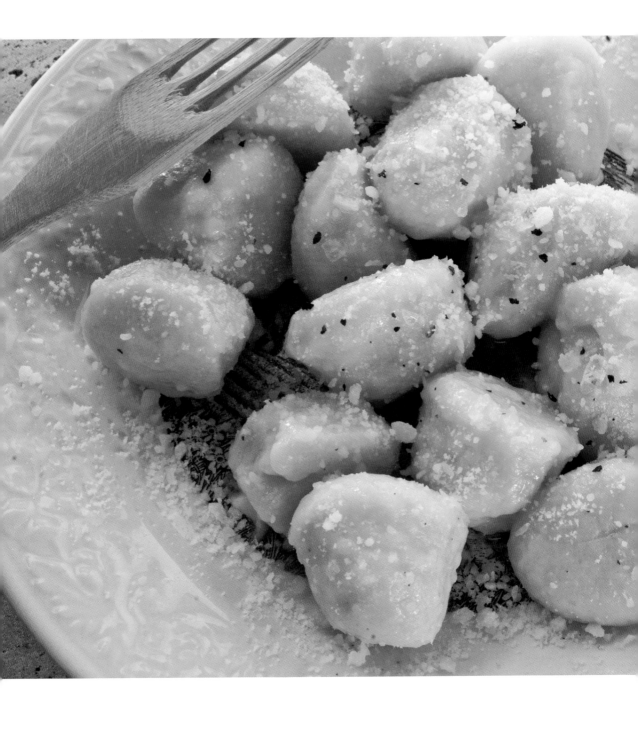

creamy risotto-style brown rice with spring greens and asiago

{ PETER BERLEY }

SERVES 4-6

Try this recipe instead of risotto. It's healthy and delicious. We often make a big batch to serve when Cody's friends stay for dinner.

Sea salt or kosher salt

9 ounces mixed spring greens, such as tatsoi, baby mustard greens, lamb's quarters, and arugula (about 9 cups)

1 tablespoon extra-virgin olive oil

1 large bunch scallions or ramps (wild leeks), trimmed and thinly sliced (about 1 cup)

1 teaspoon finely chopped garlic

2¼ cups cooked brown rice, preferably basmati, from 1 cup raw rice

1 tablespoon unsalted butter

2 ounces finely grated hard Asiago cheese (about ½ cup), plus additional for serving

Freshly ground black pepper

1. Bring a large pot of water to a boil. Add about 1½ tablespoons of salt and return to a boil. Add the greens and blanch until they are just wilted, about 1 minute. Use a spider or slotted spoon to transfer the greens to a colander and let cool slightly; reserve the cooking water.

2. Press the greens to remove excess water, then transfer them to a board and chop roughly.

3. In a large skillet over medium-high heat, warm the olive oil. Add the scallions, garlic, and a pinch of salt, and cook, stirring, until softened, about 2 minutes.

4. Stir in the rice, chopped greens, butter, and 1½ cups of the reserved cooking water and cook, stirring, over medium-high heat, until the water is almost absorbed, 3 to 4 minutes. Stir in the cheese and season with salt and pepper.

Note: Do not use fresh Asiago cheese; it's unpleasant when melted in this dish.

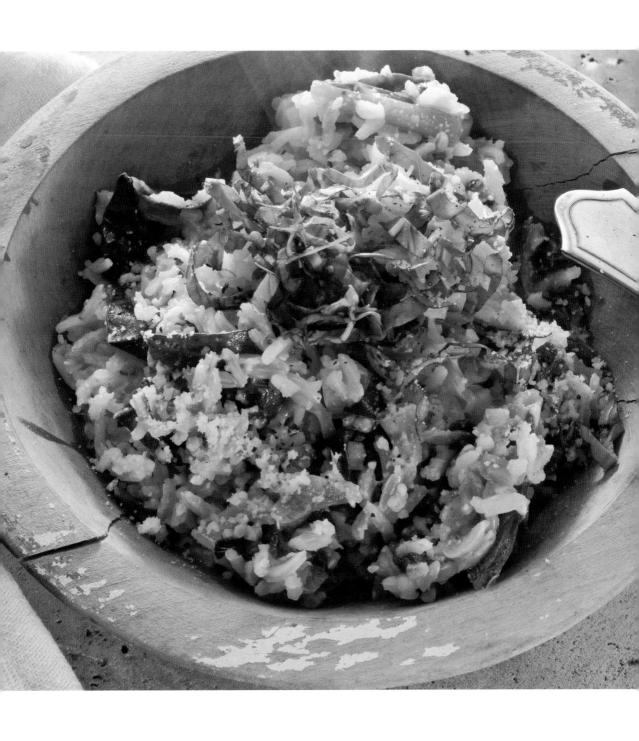

japanese pancakes

{ BARBARA LYNCH }

SERVES 4

"I make Japanese pancakes, which are a Japanese crepe almost," says Chef Barbara Lynch. "I put raw shrimp, uncooked broccoli, carrots, and kale in the batter—all raw, but it actually cooks in the pancake. I make them because they are little snacks for me, and Marchesa absolutely loves them. I think she loves them because they are round. She gets to use her chopsticks, which she loves, and we dip them in a little soy sauce. It is always fun to serve with chopsticks!" If you have pancake rings, use them to make perfect circles or other fun shapes but don't make them too thick. And if you're looking for something a bit less salty than soy sauce, try the dipping sauce I created below, which is slightly thicker and has other flavors to temper the soy sauce.

Pancakes:

1 teaspoon canola oil for skillet

1 cup all-purpose flour

½ cup water or Japanese dashi broth

1 egg

1 cup grated cabbage or pureed yam

Pinch table salt

Dash white pepper

¼ cup raw kale, stemmed and chopped small

¼ cup grated carrots

¼ cup finely chopped scallions

¼ cup boiled and chopped shrimp

Dash hot sesame oil

Pinch cumin seeds

Dipping sauce (such as a good soy sauce or make your own tangy sauce, such as Fanae's Homemade Dipping Sauce)

Fanae's Homemade Dipping Sauce:

½ cup Worcestershire sauce

¼ cup sugar

¼ cup soy sauce

¼ cup ketchup

1 tablespoon Dijon mustard

½ teaspoon ground allspice

1. Heat a skillet over medium heat. When hot, add oil.

2. Make the pancake mix by combining flour, water or dashi, egg, cabbage or yam, and salt and pepper.

3. Sprinkle the vegetables and shrimp into the batter and add sesame oil and cumin seeds (to taste).

4. Pour ¼- to ½-cup portions into the skillet. Cook pancakes, flip to finish cooking.

5. To make Fanae's Homemade Dipping Sauce, combine Worcestershire, sugar, soy sauce, and ketchup in a small saucepan. Cook over low heat, stirring, until the sugar is dissolved and the mixture reduces a bit. Stir in the mustard and allspice. Cool and serve, or store for several days, refrigerated.

6. Serve pancakes with dipping sauce.

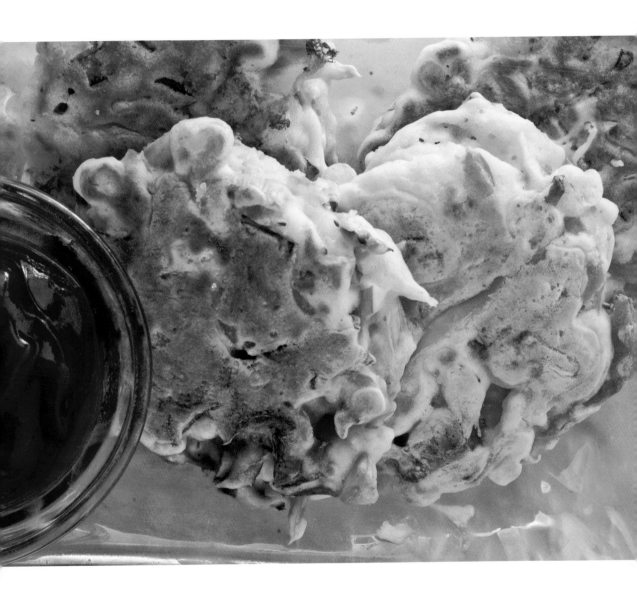

wild rice soufflé

{ DIANE FORLEY AND MICHAEL OTSUKA }

I love the exotic, earthy flavor of wild rice. Baked as a savory and sweet loaf, it is a perfect food for anyone wanting to eat whole grains and avoid gluten. You can serve this warm next to a main dish, but its flavor really comes out when it's cooled off. We eat toasted slices for breakfast when it's cold and wintry out.

5½ cups water, divided

¾ cup plus 2 tablespoons wild rice, divided

½ teaspoon salt

¼ teaspoon allspice

¼ teaspoon ground cloves

¼ teaspoon nutmeg

½ teaspoon coriander seed

2 tablespoons grits, polenta, or cornmeal (whole grain is best)

1 teaspoon butter

Salt and pepper

½ cup raisins or dried cranberries

3 eggs

1. Heat 3 cups water and ½ cup wild rice in a saucepan and bring to a boil. Add salt, turn the heat down low, and simmer, uncovered, until soft, about 45 minutes. When the wild rice is tender, drain any remaining liquid and set aside, covered, until ready to use.

2. Meanwhile, in a coffee grinder or spice mill, grind the remaining wild rice and the spices together until dry and powdery. Place in a bowl and blend in the grits, polenta, or cornmeal.

3. Heat 2½ cups water in sauce pot until just about to boil. Slowly whisk the ground wild rice mixture into the hot water. Turn the heat down to low and continue to stir intermittently until the mixture thickens into a porridge, about 20 minutes. Turn off the heat and stir in butter. Season with salt and pepper and taste, adding more salt if necessary; it should taste a tiny bit salty.

4. Pour the porridge mixture into a large bowl and mix in the cooked wild rice. (This mixture can be stored in the fridge to continue the next day.)

5. Preheat oven to 375°F and thoroughly butter a medium-size loaf pan.

6. Add the raisins or cranberries to the wild rice mixture and stir to combine.

7. Separate the eggs, placing the whites in a medium-size metal bowl and the yolks in a small bowl. Beat the yolks with a hand mixer on high or whisk until thick and pale, about 3 minutes, and then, using clean beaters, beat the whites on high until they have soft, glossy peaks, about 2 minutes.

8. Gradually mix egg yolks into the wild rice mixture, stirring throughout, then fold in beaten egg whites.

9. Scrape into the buttered loaf pan and bake until a toothpick comes out clean and the soufflé is browned on top, about 60 minutes. Remove from the oven and let rest for 5 to 10 minutes. With a knife, loosen the soufflé from around the edges of the pan before removing. The soufflé can be served warm or, once cool, stored in plastic wrap.

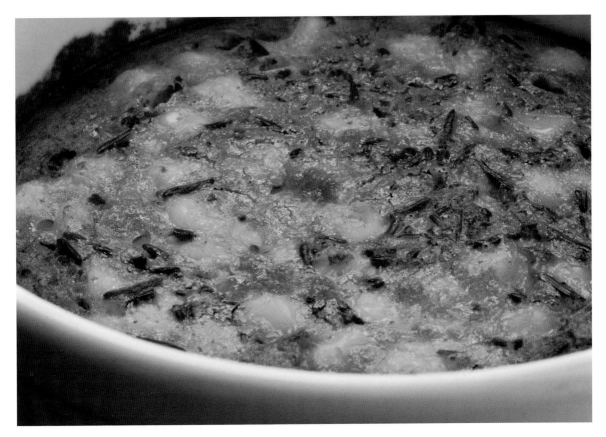

savory waffles

{ LINTON HOPKINS }

SERVES 4

"One thing my kids really love," says Chef Linton Hopkins, "is when it's raining outside at lunchtime and we make a batch of savory waffles. Instead of sugar and syrup, we just fold in Parmesan and Gruyère, if I have some sitting in the refrigerator, and salt and pepper. We use that as a complement to a bunch of soups, like tomato soup. We have a waffle iron that has shapes of animals and a barn, so I ask my kids, 'Do you want to be the pig today? Or the chicken? Or have a cow?'" If you have some sliced ham, you can fold the waffle and make a fun ham sandwich with the waffle as the perfect crispy bun, and in springtime you can add sautéed and chopped asparagus to the batter.

Try adding herbs and other seasonal produce, like pumpkin puree, to the batter instead of cheese. Hopkins makes his waffles from scratch, but you can use your favorite ready mix. We like the multigrain mix from Bob's Red Mill.

2 cups waffle and pancake mix

2 eggs

2 cups milk

2 tablespoons vegetable oil

Salt and pepper

¾ cup grated good Parmesan cheese

½ cup grated Gruyère or similar cheese

1. Preheat oven to 200°F and place a waiting plate to warm inside. Heat a waffle maker until a flick of water beads and bounces around.

2. Prepare the waffle mix, adding eggs, milk, oil, salt, and pepper, and mix until just combined, adding more milk if the mix is too thick. It should be the consistency of pudding. Then fold in the cheeses.

3. Lightly butter the waffle maker and spoon judicious dollops of the mix onto the center of the hot waffle iron and spread just a bit. The mix will spread when the lid closes and expand as it cooks, so adding too much will be a bit messy as it bubbles out the sides.

4. As the waffles finish, use a fork to lift them off and put them in the oven to stay warm while the rest are made. Waffles are best served warm. Freeze any leftover waffles to enjoy later.

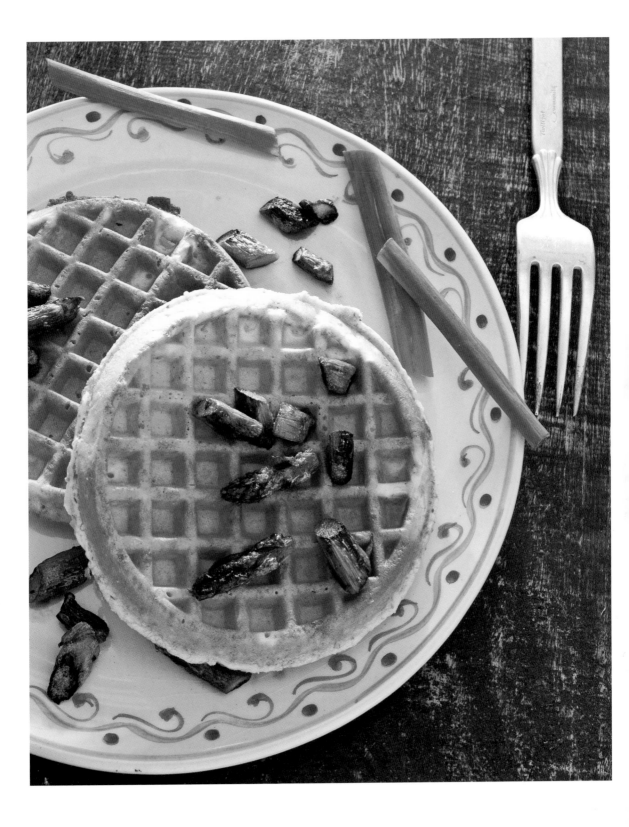

chickpea panisse with carrot ginger butter

{ PETER BERLEY }

SERVES 4

Peter Berley says *panisses* are a perfect snack for kids. Spread with the Carrot Ginger Butter and topped with toasted almonds, they are especially delicious. You can also simply dust them with sugar or for adults sprinkle them with salt and cracked black pepper. Sometimes we add cardamom and cinnamon while the chickpea flour is cooking, and mix in a teaspoon of honey before it cools.

You can make fingers and bake them as below or cut into rounds. You can also try frying them in ½ inch of hot oil (put them in when snakelike patterns appear in the oil). Whichever way you decide to make them, serve right away.

Panisses:

1 cup chickpea flour

2⅔ cups cold water

¾ teaspoon salt

3 tablespoons butter

Vegetable oil

1 tablespoon olive oil

½ teaspoon salt

⅓ cup sliced almonds (optional)

Carrot Ginger Butter:

12 ounces carrots, peeled and thinly sliced

2 cups plus 1 tablespoon water, divided

2 teaspoons peeled and finely chopped ginger

¼ teaspoon sea salt

1 tablespoon honey or light brown sugar

1 tablespoon lemon juice

Sea salt and freshly ground white pepper

1. To make the panisses, combine the chickpea flour and water in a bowl and whisk until smooth. Strain the mixture through a strainer into a heavy medium saucepan to remove any lumps. Add the salt and butter and cook over high heat, whisking continuously, until the mixture is smooth and thick. Reduce the heat as low as possible and simmer, covered, for 20 minutes.

2. Uncover and whisk again until smooth. Pour into a 7 x 11-inch baking dish or a 10-inch pie plate and refrigerate until set (about 40 minutes). This can be done up to 3 days ahead. Store in the refrigerator sealed with plastic wrap.

3. Meanwhile, begin making the Carrot Ginger Butter by combining carrots, 2 cups water, ginger, salt, and honey or brown sugar in a pan and simmering, covered, until tender. Uncover the pan and cook until liquid has evaporated.

4. Preheat oven to 375°F.

5. Transfer the carrot mixture to a food processor, add the lemon juice and 1 tablespoon water, and puree. Season with salt and white pepper.

6. Lightly brush a heavy baking sheet with vegetable oil. Spread the sliced almonds on a separate ungreased baking sheet and toast in the oven for about 7 minutes, watching carefully so they don't burn and stirring once midway.

7. Meanwhile, run a thin knife around the edge of the panisse and unmold onto a cutting surface. Slice into bite-size squares or rectangles or cut with cookie cutters. Transfer the shapes to a large bowl and brush (or gently toss) them with 1 tablespoon olive oil.

8. Spread the panisses over the prepared baking sheet and bake for 20 minutes until crisp and golden.

9. After cooling slightly, spread each with Carrot Ginger Butter, top with the toasted almonds, and serve immediately.

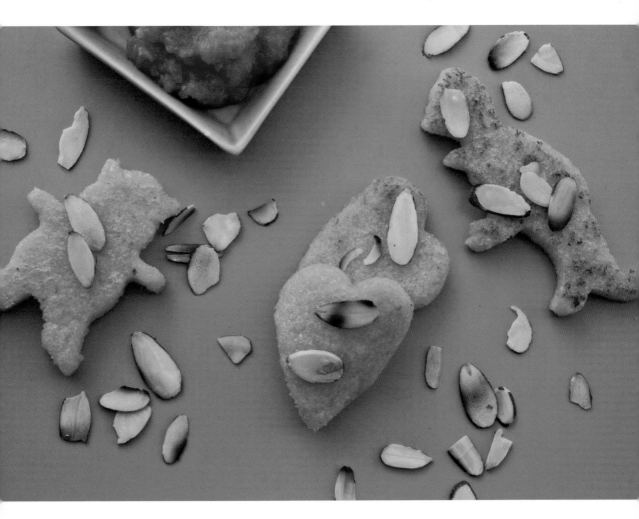

adolescence

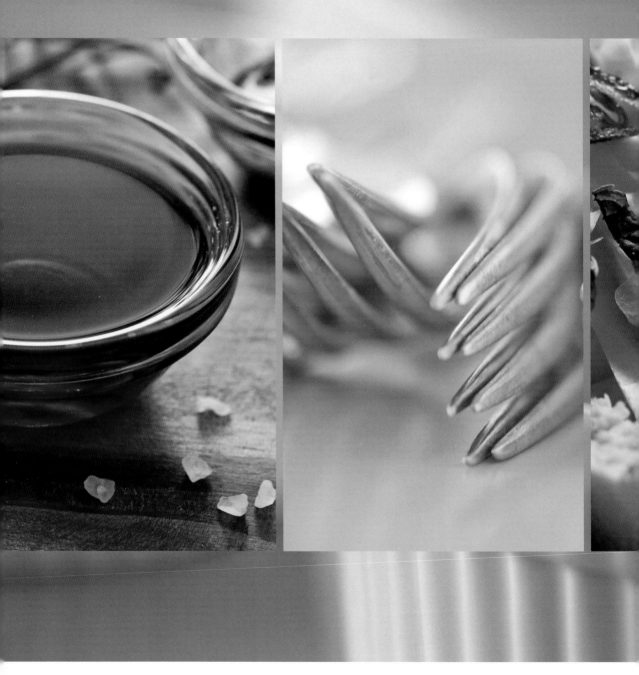

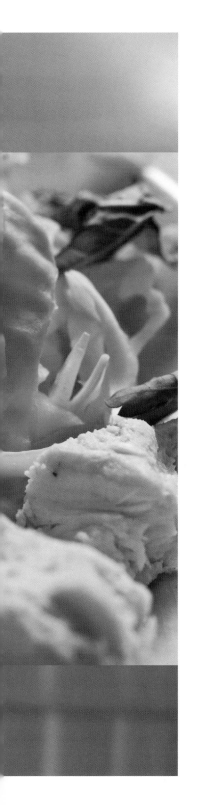

THINKING AND EATING FOR THEMSELVES

ages eight to eleven

Eric Bromberg, chef and co-owner of New York City's Blue Ribbon restaurants, says that at this age his kids will try almost anything. His children are as curious and bold as he is about tasting different foods, though they still initially display the kind of hesitancy and trepidation that most kids will. Most of the chefs I interviewed have cultivated a culinary curiosity and openness in their children, and their children easily and confidently rattle off their likes and dislikes, their knowledge about ingredients, and even simple cooking strategies. They can instantly discern quality and freshness and articulate it in detail. Bromberg's son, Jason, says excitedly that he likes when chicken is roasted with mushrooms tucked under the skin.

When his children were younger, Floyd Cardoz, chef at New York's Tabla Restaurant, embraced cooking more traditional family meals. At their present ages he cooks an extensive repertoire at home for family meals, including pasta with truffles and osso bucco, and even interesting side dishes like a salad with pine nuts, olives, and anchovies.

Focusing on Nutrition

The focus of all chefs with children this age is trying to manage nutritional balance for their children. At eight, children are still moody about food and go through phases of coveting favorite foods.

"It's important to recognize the parents' role in teaching and educating the kids about food, about society and social aspects," says Alexandria chef Cathal Armstrong. "I really try to maintain that they eat a balanced diet—some proteins, some carbohydrates, some vitamins, some minerals. Just consider a balanced diet and not worry too much about 'Well, we had broccoli yesterday, we can't have broccoli again today.' If it's a vegetable they like and will eat, give them more of it."

Armstrong's daughter, Eve, who was a hesitant eater during her preschool years, now enjoys a broad culinary repertoire. She especially loves eating fish and meat. Favorite family dinners include roast chicken, roast pork, and ribs. Armstrong says she is still at times reluctant to try new foods, but a patient approach does eventually bring her around.

> "My children have a really good relationship with food—that's the point. They know how to enjoy it, they know how to prepare it for themselves, and I'm just really grateful for that. The legacy I can leave them is that you can really nourish yourself."
>
> —Peter Berley, New York City chef and award-winning cookbook author

Both of Josiah Citrin's children pick through their meals, separating and reassembling what's on their plate for themselves. Citrin, chef and owner of Los Angeles restaurant Melisse, considers himself lucky, though, saying, "My kids like eating healthy things—they like eating broccoli, they eat carrots, and they eat salad every night." His approach is to give them the foods they like to eat, like Mexican food or Korean food, but to make sure the foods are flavored authentically and not Americanized, and also that they're made with quality ingredients.

"Real food's the most important thing," says Linton Hopkins, chef and owner of Atlanta's Restaurant Eugene. "I don't change the way I think about food—being at home or being in the restaurant." His approach is to get ingredients both local and fresh, putting them together in simple ways. Flavor comes from the ingredients he selects, enhanced with careful preparation and the addition of simple sauces. The food is regionally traditional in its ingredients and made from scratch.

About cooking at home for his family, Hopkins says, "I really don't try to 'gussy up' the food by putting too many ingredients in—as a professional cook, I've learned that more and more I'm pulling items out of a dish and making a recipe that's under five ingredients—I'm just trying to select the best of those ingredients. So that roast chicken really tastes like roast chicken. I just maybe squeeze some lemon on it at the table; I use citrus fruit a lot in cooking because we want to have that good acid balance." Roasting a chicken is easy, and he says, "I think my total prep time on roasting a chicken is about two minutes. I turn on the oven and put a chicken in an iron skillet with salt and roast it for forty-five minutes."

Hopkins speaks warmly of growing up with home-cooked meals prepared by both his mother and his grandfather, Eugene. Chef and cookbook author Peter Berley expresses a similar sentiment when he says, "What became the most important thing was eating together as much as possible—we were completely dedicated to eating dinner together. That was like a rock—we ate dinner together all the time, every night." Every chef I interviewed agrees: Family time at this age is important, and so is eating well together.

It's much easier to get your kids to sit at the table and eat, and to eat well, if you started when they were young. If you started at the beginning, feeding them vegetables, talking to them about healthy foods, and sitting with them together at meals, then at this age, these things are part of their routine.

Healthy Strategies for Picky Eaters

Citrin says that at his house, his wife limits after-school snacks and then will steam broccoli for their children before dinner. "We always start them off with the vegetables before as an appetizer, so they eat them when they're hungry," he says.

Chef Jimmy Schmidt did start early feeding his children healthy foods, but his oldest son, Michael

Blu, is still a picky eater. Schmidt, chef at Rattlesnake restaurants in the Midwest, attributes this to his highly developed sense of smell. "So to a foreign smell, his immediate response is, 'this is weird.'" Of the vegetables he likes, he prefers them raw to cooked. "I'll be making dinner, and he'll come in and say 'That's stinky. It smells like rotten eggs. He's right—there are sulfides in asparagus." Sulfides are also in broccoli, cabbage, onions, peppers, cauliflower, brussels sprouts, rutabagas, and turnips. "It's been tricky since he was a baby," say Schmidt. "He didn't like pureed peas or other vegetable purees. He'll eat cooked carrots, but he prefers them raw; most vegetables he prefers raw. Cauliflower is blander, and I'll use purple and orange cauliflower, which he thinks is cool looking."

Citrin says of his children, "They weren't as picky in the beginning, and then they got picky." Augustin, Citrin's son, will taste anything in the kitchen while playing chef in the restaurant during the prep hours, but it's hard to get him to eat a whole meal, says Citrin. But Augustin likes the artichoke soup at the restaurant, as well as the crab cakes and the onion soup. He also likes caviar and sautéed *foie gras* with pineapple—a gourmet treat that is undoubtedly a perk of owning a restaurant.

Both of Citrin's children enjoy eating salads, broccoli, carrots, turkey sausages, and pea soup, but neither likes cooked tomatoes. He incorporates foods they like into new dishes with other foods, and he cooks at-home variations of dishes they like from their weekly outing to their favorite local Korean barbecue restaurant. Citrin says, "That's why I eat at Manpuku once a week. They eat everything. He loves

that place. He eats the beef. I don't know what it is about that place." There his son adores the seaweed salad, the avocado rolls. He loves the daikon and purple carrot salad so much that the waiters bring him a plate of it as soon as they see him coming in the door.

Fitting in with Food

This is an age where friends are important, and so is fitting in and being cool. It's an age of secret codes and inside jokes and made-up languages, and kids have a strong need to belong. Eating cool things is part of that, and no kid wants to feel weird. Virant says he doesn't want his children to go to a friend's house and feel like they are the "weird" kids because they don't eat what their friends eat. "Food's kind of a cool thing. And my oldest daughter just did a report for class on Japan and food in Japan. She did it on her own, and at first she was kind of embarrassed and scared because she thought all the other kids were gonna think it's gross to eat octopus and fish eggs. It turned out everybody liked it—her eyes were opened, and she was like, 'Wow, that was really cool!'"

Bromberg thinks his openness in allowing his children to eat freely what they like "promotes them to eat other things that they may be hesitant about trying" He says he prefers his children not to eat things like candy, but, "I think it's pretty complicated, especially when your kid isn't with you all the time and candy is available. I think it just creates a really weird relationship." It's a trade-off, he says.

Bromberg calls himself an experimental eater, and his kids have learned to follow suit. "We'll go to Chinatown and they'll eat jellyfish," he says of his children. "I mean, some things they'll spit out and say that was disgusting, but they'll try just about anything." Jason, Bromberg's son, tells me, "Sometimes, the best thing is the thing that looks horrible." He mentions asparagus as an example of something he initially thought of as "ew" but turned out to be "really good." "It seemed like that seaweed soup was disgusting, but then when I tried it, it was delicious," he adds. Bromberg explains that the first time, Jason didn't try the soup at all. Then the second time he did try and decided it was pretty cool. Bromberg says, "We order anything, and I'm as adventurous as I can be. I love everything about food and cultures. Whenever we go somewhere, we try and focus on the foods that are native to that region. We're in a restaurant that's on the ocean, so we should have things that come from here that are in the ocean, and likewise when you're at a Holiday Inn in Iowa, you don't necessarily want to have the shrimp cocktail!"

Exposing his children to real eating is important, and he says, "Maybe it's silly, from an economic point of view, but if they want to eat a lobster when we're out to dinner at a restaurant, we let them order a lobster, and the three children share it." He says, "If that makes it a positive dining experience in a restaurant for them, then it makes more sense to me than if they have the kids' hamburger and fries or fried chicken fingers and fries."

Palates expand with age, and Schmidt's son continues to open up to new foods. Schmidt helps that process along. He says, "I use different types of sea salt for different dishes. I also use flavored sea salts

with herbs and stuff in them. My children don't pick up on it, but they are getting a broader flavor profile." Schmidt says of Michael Blu, "As he gets older, he learns to navigate his senses better. His eating will expand when he's able to assimilate unusual smells or new smells and associate them with foods that actually taste good to his palate, like fish. We don't put any pressure on it." Schmidt says Michael Blu is "setting his own pace on how he's expanding his food." He will try foods his friends like to eat and will come home asking for foods his friends say they like eating. At this age kids are acutely aware of what is going on with their friends and classmates. "It's his opportunity," says Schmidt, who makes sure those opportunities are taken advantage of. "I do collect their feedback, like with Michael on his aroma issue. You got to look at it from his perspective—is there something else here that's triggering this effect? Then I try to expose them to new things."

Engage Kids in the Process and Preparation

Making the kitchen the family zone is a good way to engage kids with cooking, too. Even limited partici-pation connects them to the food. "Usually they're doing their homework right there on the sort of bar/ ledge next to the stovetop and see us cooking," says Hopkins. "I made a curry, and Avery wasn't a huge fan of the smell, but she actually liked the flavor."

Buying fruits and vegetables at the store is not as deeply gratifying and rewarding as picking them yourself. Being out in a field, seeing how vegetables grow and picking them yourself, is a way to open kids

JIMMY SCHMIDT is a three-time James Beard Award winner and owner of the Rattlesnake Club restaurants in Denver and Detroit. Celebrated chef, restaurateur, food scientist, and innovator, he focuses on traditional cooking methods to create simple, rustic, and healthy dishes. His numerous awards include the James Beard Award for Best Chef Midwest, *Wine Spectator*'s Award of Excellence and *Gourmet* magazine's America's Top Tables and America's Best Restaurants. Schmidt is also involved in developing nutritional products for athletes who need to eat efficiently for stamina and focus and has his own products, LifeForceV and Life2Go. He has also served as the director of sports nutrition for GM/Corvette Racing and has coordinated catering services for the "24 Hours of Le Mans" race in France since 1999. He is the father of three boys: Michael Blu, Jasse Sonic, and Cadet Bar. He says of feeding his family, "The big thing at the end of the day is that food is seasonal and as pure as possible—it's not manufactured—it doesn't have ingredients in it that you don't know what they are."

Jimmy Schmidt : MARSHALL WILLIAMS

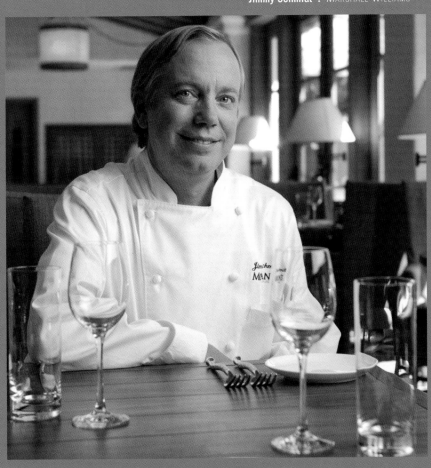

JOSIAH CITRIN uniquely crafts his menu at Melisse, his refined French restaurant in Santa Monica, with seasonal finds from the local farmers' market. He left an early career as a tournament surfer to travel to France and learn to cook. Melisse earned two stars from the Michelin guide, #1 for Top Food in Los Angeles (2006, 2008, 2009) and #1 American-French Restaurant for Food in Los Angeles (2003–2010) by Zagat Guide, Four Stars by Mobile Travel Guide (2001–2009), *Wine Spectator* Best Award of Excellence (2001–2008), and Top 40 Restaurants by Gayot .com since 2006. Citrin has a son, Augustin, and a younger daughter, Olivia. Augustin has a discerning palate and can be vocal about his disappointments. Citrin finds himself teaching life lessons like, "When the bacon's overcooked, it's overcooked, it is what it is—part of life." He says, "I wait for the day when I can go to a 2-star and 3-star restaurant in France with my kids. Or a bistro and order *tete de veau*—I think I will get that day with them, they'll get there."

Josiah Citrin in the kitchen at Melisse : MARY ANN MARINO

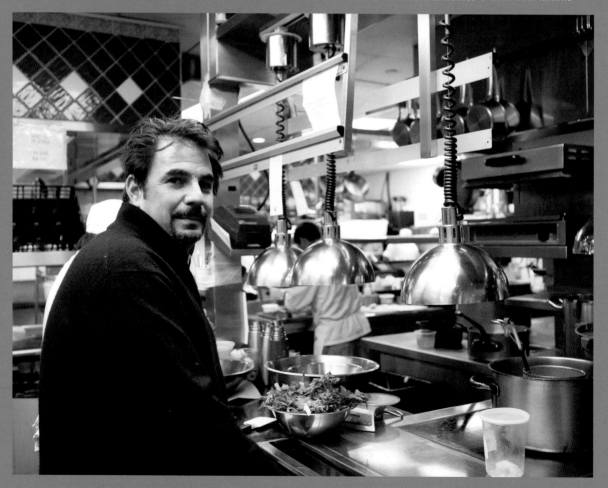

up about vegetables so they become more than foods on a plate they are being pestered to eat. A small child might try spinach and other greens if told those foods are what make their favorite superhero strong, but older children need more intellectual stimulation and hands-on involvement. Schmidt tells a story about when Michael Blu visited his grandparents who live in Northern Michigan, where he went wild-blueberry picking. While he liked blueberries before, his earthy experience picking them himself made them more delectable. They also go every fall as a family to local orchards to pick apples. They eat them right there off the tree, crisp and sweet. "We try to hit as many local farms to experience it. We go to different farmers' markets to see different fruits and vegetables and they try things."

Virant makes a ritual winter jaunt into the forest with his children to see the sugar maple trees tapped for making maple syrup. They hear a naturalist talk about the syrup-making process and visit a little hut to see sap for the syrup boiling down in an iron kettle over a crackling wood fire. At home, they make hot cereal and use that syrup.

Simple Home Cooking

Hopkins says the methods of home cooking are a lot simpler than cooking in his restaurant. He explains the difference this way: "At Restaurant Eugene, we'd take a chicken and make chicken four ways on the same plate—we'd get the breast that we would have sautéed and then bring it up in like a bucket poach, and then we'd have the skin that we'd take off and recrisp so we'd have a sheath of chicken crackling,

and then we'd make confit from the leg to pack in ravioli, and then we'd have a reduction of sauce from the bones and the gizzards and the liver that would be the sauce. So, it's a much different intent at home; I'm not going for that kind of flavor. At home you don't have that team of cooks and that time, so at home it's being able to know how to roast a chicken." He says, "I really don't spend more than thirty minutes. Roast chicken, for example: It's two minutes to get that chicken in the oven. I know that the meal itself will take forty-five minutes, but to put on a pot of rice, to get the chicken roasting in the oven, and then clean the salad greens and have a vinaigrette, my total prep time is probably twelve minutes. And then I just wait for the chicken and the rice to finish and then plate up is another five."

He explains his methods: "What we'll do at home is take the roast chicken and we'll eat all the meat off in one night. Then I'll make a stock from those bones while I'm cleaning up from dinner, and then we'll have chicken soup and rice the next day. So, we try to make things using methods to get multiple meals from one item and not have a culture of throwing foods away. My kids love how when we buy a roasting chicken, we'll pull the liver out and just fry that up and eat the liver. They see us do it first—we don't throw it away. I really don't think of a food as gross, in its raw state—and my kids see that philosophy around food; they are raised in our culture of food. So instead of using just the bottoms of the leeks, we use the tops and make a leek broth. And then we incorporate the stocks as much as we can. We incorporate the

"The refined carbohydrates (white pasta, white rice, white bread, or anything made with refined white flour or white sugar) are not very nutritious—they're not good for you. Technically what they do is spike your blood sugar to high levels that cause your body to dump insulin into your bloodstream. Your blood sugar spikes first, then crashes. There's no doubt gyrations in blood sugar and insulin are the source for diabetes—a great concern.

"At this age my children are so active, they are not storing fat, any of them—they are converting all their food into running around and growing. My kids are super lean. My focus is getting the protein and the carbs in them because they're so active. Protein should be an important part of kids' diets—meat, eggs, dairy, cheese, chicken, steaks, roasted pork. But if you look at what kids eat—the pizza, the pasta, the french fries—you start to add up a whole lot of carbs and not a lot of protein. It is also relative to their mood, their energy levels, and how often they get colds and get sick. Amino acids are the building blocks of proteins; they're real essential nutrient components that kids can't always assimilate in food easily, especially if they have picky diets.

"Trying to get everything in your bloodstream to fire most efficiently is pretty hard to do. Balanced blood sugar is essential, and the low glycemic index is the more stable environment for it. Kids have more stable energy too when they eat low-glycemic foods—they don't run into crashes, or mood swings. For Le Mans, where they have twenty-four-hours-straight car racing, I do their whole menu to specifically keep them away from refined carbs, because if you see a driver eat a candy bar after he's been up fourteen or sixteen hours, his blood sugar spikes, insulin kicks in, and he will be sleeping over a tire, and it will kill him.

"When I cook at home, if I use butter, I use really good butter, but everything is in moderation. I cook a lot of things in olive oil. I use jellies that are made with cane syrup instead of high-fructose corn syrup, and I use organic peanut butter. My kids eat a reasonable amount of whole-protein pastas like those from Bionature. Sometimes I add in vegetables; I'll julienne the zucchini so it looks like the pasta, just a different color. At the end of the day, the big picture is that I'm serving food to my children that is seasonal, as pure as possible, and not manufactured—it doesn't come from a box and have ingredients in it that you don't know what they are."

stocks in everyday cooking—I really believe that helps with flavor."

To make the stock, he says, you take the leftover roast chicken and bones and you put it in a pot with just enough water to barely cover it, and you've got a stock in an hour. When cooking at home, he says he thinks about making things spicy that he likes but his children are hesitant about. "If I do a sauté like a stir-fry of chicken, I'll put fresh peppers like serranos or little Vietnamese chiles on the side for my wife, Gina, and me to fold into our meal. We do put Tabasco and Crystal hot sauce on the table, which my children love putting on their eggs. We want them to start slowly in adding that sense to their taste."

Bromberg takes a similar approach to home cooking. He says, too, that he cooks simple things at home and mentions roast chicken and sautéed spinach. Some nights he says are just vegetarian—good rice and beans or grains. About roast chicken, he says, "It's the simplest thing to do, and it's not like red meat, where it has to be cooked properly and it's no good when it's reheated. Also, you can make an awful lot of things out of a roast chicken! And if you have it already cooked, it's a breeze."

Hopkins says, "Mostly at home it's vegetables as a side dish. So it'll be this tomato fondue, and then there'll be a big sauté of some bok choy we picked up at the market, and then there'll be a bowl of rice and then our protein and then maybe a little sauce."

One way chefs manage to cook their meals so efficiently is by having some foods prepped and ready to go. Hopkins says, "It's really trying to roll your basic prep into multiple meals. . . . Sometimes we'll

roast a chicken, and that'll become chicken salad. Or that leftover roast chicken becomes shredded into a pasta the next day." That kind of cooking comes from experience. It saves time because meals are not started from scratch, and it is much more economical. Starting meals from scratch every day is not only time-consuming, but it's also much more expensive.

I was given the *Joy of Cooking* as a gift by my mother-in-law when I first got married, but I didn't cook much then. I learned to cook when we had Cody and became a family. Family cooking is a much different sport than cooking for, say, a dinner party or a meal for two at home. Learning from the chefs interviewed in this book, I am a much more efficient cook, and I see beyond one meal in my cooking. I buy and make a whole chicken instead of just the breast or thigh so that I can have leftovers. I am creative with prepped foods and use them as ready ingredients in making meals, and don't just reheat the same dish the next day, which nobody really wants. When I do buy just chicken breasts, I buy and cook a couple of extra.

Hopkins also cooks strategically. "For example, when we make tomato sauce, we'll make a big batch that's enough for two or three meals, and then we can freeze leftovers if we don't want to eat it the next day," he says. Dinner in the summertime is fast, he says, because, "we're really out on the grill a lot."

It's true that cooking fish or steak on the grill can be very easy and fast. Lots of chefs mentioned using the grill to cook summertime meals. If you're starting with very fresh fish or meat, it takes only a bit of seasoning and technique to make it delicious. Hopkins says he also resorts to simple things like a

FLOYD CARDOZ was born in Bombay and is executive chef and co-owner with restaurateur Danny Meyer of Tabla in New York City. He is the author of *One Spice, Two Spice*, where he shares many personal stories and his unique cross-cultural blend of Indian and French cuisines. He has two sons, Justin and Peter. He says of dinners at home, "We always have greens with our meals, like a few weeks ago I made osso bucco—real osso bucco. But I couldn't figure out how to get the vegetables in it because the dish was so different, so I made a green bean salad. I know my kids love olives and pine nuts, so I put olives and pine nuts and anchovies in the salad, and they enjoyed it."

baked potato and salad night. He lists risotto and stir-fries as other simple family meals that he loves making at home. He says, "My wife doesn't like when we do breakfast for dinner, but occasionally I love that. I've got some bacon and eggs lying around and some toast, so it can be very quick!"

Citrin says he keeps *queso fresco,* the Mexican cheese, around that his children like. He makes a quick meal of corn tortillas with rice and beans, some chicken, and the queso fresco. I make tacos for Cody and myself for dinner out of almost anything—leftover slow-roasted beef is very satisfying in a taco.

Also, it's worth investing in some simple tools to help with prep. A proper cutting knife that is sharp will be a lot faster to use when chopping vegetables like carrots or potatoes than struggling with a small paring knife. Hopkins says, "The speed that professional cooks work at is unknown at home. . . . I can clean/break down an entire kitchen at home in ten minutes. All dishes, all done, in the dishwasher, sink clean, oven wiped down, done." While sometimes I like the slow meandering pace of cooking and cleaning after a hectic day, I learned from Hopkins that when I am focused and organized, I can be much faster and more efficient at getting meals cooked, dishes done, and all put away. Sometimes, it works out that I can clean everything up the last ten minutes while dinner is cooking and before I even put out the food.

Eating One Family Meal

Schedules are hectic at this age. Citrin admits that his date night with his wife and his son's guitar lessons have interrupted the ritual of their special Monday cooking nights. At every age the family dinner table changes, but all the chefs interviewed for this book agree about the importance of sharing meals and social time together. "I have breakfast or lunch together with my daughter every Tuesday. I take her to John O'Groats," says Citrin. They also have ritual weekly family outings to Manpuku, their favorite local Korean barbecue.

At home, even though eating preferences can differ for every member of the family, it is more important than ever at this age to share a collective, if not a cohesive, meal. "We try to find the perfect meal for our kids as opposed to saying 'this is our family meal,'" says Armstrong. Meals that work for

"I remember celebrity chef Jacques Pepin saying that he didn't have any food rules at the table, but you know, as a parent, how can you have that? There is always some kind of rule that comes out of your mouth. A big rule is what ingredients are allowed in the house—that seems to be the biggest rule. And before you get seconds in anything, you have to have eaten everything at least once. You have to eat that first plate completely. Also, you can't leave the table until you've tried at least two bites of everything. They may eat just five or seven bites of something and they're done, the portions are smaller. Look at the size of their stomachs, they're just smaller. Also, the kids set the table. That's a thing in our house. They have to get the napkins, the glasses of water, and the knife and fork. Gina, my wife, teaches them about it—what side the fork and the knife and the spoon go on. You can't just throw the napkin on the table at the place setting; it goes on a certain area on the place setting. There are so many lessons around the table that are just great. No one just dives in until we say a little blessing together. Thanks for our food, and then we begin. We pass and share, and that's the sort of culture we want to teach our children."

everyone can be constructed by using simple strategies like serving sauces and condiments on the side and offering foods family style so each person can select the foods she prefers.

"The whole attitude of 'I don't want that for dinner' is off-limits at our house. . . . They get input. We'll talk about it ahead of time, when we go to the farmers' market on a certain day, and we'll give them some money, and they'll go pick some things up so they're proud to bring home those vegetables that they bought. And I think that's a great way to include them in the choices," says Hopkins. "Our priority is making sure they're included in the raw food choices, like, 'Hey! Do you want to have spinach tonight or asparagus?' We frame it in a question like that."

Armstrong agrees and says, "I think it's important to feed kids what they want to eat." He says his kids enjoy eating vegetables because he initially introduced them patiently in small amounts.

Cooking with and for Kids

Chefs' kids begin cooking for themselves through curiosity. They see their parents playfully mixing, combining, and tasting, and they want to do it, too. They experiment: "Why don't we just take a little of this and a little of that . . . this is how you cook. I've learned that cooking is what happens between the lines of a recipe. If you just put me in a space with ingredients, I'm gonna come up with forms and shapes from those ingredients," says Hopkins. And he adds, "I find having a sauce in your food really helps. You know, a little pan drippings left over from the roast chicken to put on your rice. I'll make simple little meals like chicken with mushrooms and will bring the stock around and actually create a sauce."

His daughter, Avery, at eight years old enjoys sauces on her foods, too, to spread on and to dip into, and she began making her own concoctions. "Avery calls it 'cobbydo'—a little sauce she made," says Hopkins. "I just let her go to the refrigerator with a little ramekin and she makes a soy, Worcestershire, and mustard mayonnaise. Because it has soy in it, she calls it a 'Chinese cobbydo. . . .' We'll have roast chicken, so she'll dip her chicken into it, and it's really good! It's great with fish; you can use it on salmon, too."

And his son tries new things with food, too. "There was a period with my son where'd he'd just chop everything up together and mix it into this weird mash, a horrible looking . . . indescribable thing," Hopkins explains. "He did it once with a Mexican meal with tortillas. It turned into something horrid, and he couldn't eat it. We teach him not to just junk it up too much on the plate."

Hopkins believes in foraging for the best ingredients and then cooking them simply. "I'm an ingredient-based cook, and we try to really be an ingredient-based household," he says. To teach his kids, he says, "We don't go the store with recipes, saying, 'This is what we have to get.' We have certain staples and go-tos, our vegetables, and our meat, and bread we get from our own bakery. Let's just get the good ingredients in the house and then we'll just cook. If I have a little flour and cornmeal around, we'll make little johnnycakes, or maybe I'll just have cornmeal and fold in a little butter to it. I always have buttermilk in my refrigerator—it's a great thing for the whole world of quick breads and for folding into soups. Kids love little pancakes and quick breads—they are always a hit. So we have cast-iron skillets and griddles going all the time. I'll have some ground pork, and we'll have citrus fruit, always, on hand. I love having mustards and coating chicken before it goes on the grill. Buttermilk's always a great marinade. We really try to celebrate the ingredients."

An important role parents can play in that part of their children's education is to get them to participate in meal preparation. "I always get the kids involved in making the dinner," says Armstrong. "Picking the herbs, peeling the garlic, chopping the garlic, and things like that—with a garlic crusher, not with a knife; they are not ready for knives yet. I think it's really important to be involved in the preparation of the meal and the cleanup of the meal, because it develops good habits and good sensibilities in general," he says.

Josiah Citrin adds, "When I make fish with breading or something, then it's good 'cause my children can help me do it." Bromberg points out that stoves are awkward things for kids even at this age, and he tries to do things away from the stove.

"One of the tremendous things about the kids participating in cooking is the participation starts with this comment: 'Turn the television off. Let's go work in the kitchen,'" says Armstrong. "Just get them to participate in something with their mother or father, just that part itself, is really important."

What's a "No"?

"Nothing's a 'no'—not even McDonald's," says Citrin. "It's a balancing act, and I don't want to have any no's, because no's just lead to—sneaky." His approach has been to build a repertoire of healthy foods his children enjoy, like Dover sole with lemon; lemon chicken that he broils; pork cutlets with lemon on them, a particular favorite; and turkey chili.

LINTON HOPKINS opened Restaurant Eugene, named for his grandfather, with his wife, Gina, who is the restaurant sommelier, in 2004. His menu reflects his strong ties to local farmers, with dishes that combine his traditional Southern upbringing with formal French techniques and showcase his knack for culinary experimentation. He was one of *Food & Wine*'s Best New Chefs in 2009 and was also nominated in 2009 for a James Beard Award for Best Chef Southeast. He is the father of a son, Linton, and a daughter, Avery. He says of his children, "They are raised in our culture of food, that's how they think about it. You know, they take the lead from us without a doubt. . . . Of course, in our household, we talk a lot about food."

Linton and Gina Hopkins, daughter Avery, and son Linton : BEALL & THOMAS PHOTOGRAPHY

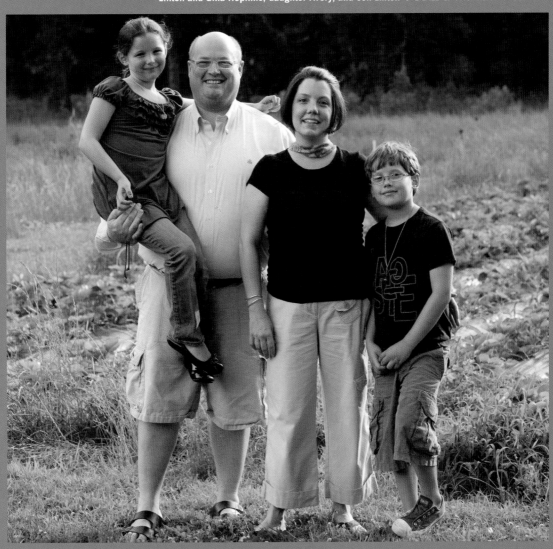

Sally Kravich, a natural health expert, says, "When people tell me what they are craving, I find out what they are missing nutritionally." For example, if your child craves salt, that's an indicator that he is not getting enough vegetables in his diet. If she craves fats like cheese or avocado, then she is not getting enough fatty acids in her diet. If children crave cheese and dairy, they need more calcium. She adds that sugar in the diet ensures children will be more nervous.

Fast food is a big issue for chefs' families. It embodies the antithesis of the kinds of food and appreciation for food that they embrace. "We need to know about why we don't go to McDonald's," says Hopkins. "I love cheeseburgers, so I'll cook cheeseburgers at home. I don't believe cheeseburgers are bad for you. Good meat and real cheese and bakery bread, that's good for you. I teach that distinction about what is bad food and what is good food."

Armstong says of his children, "Their friends go to McDonald's, and my children say, you know, we just don't eat that. I would tell them, don't be rude about it; there's no reason to be offensive about it—my children just won't eat anything that comes from McDonald's. They know what's in it, they know what the truth is, and they won't eat it."

It's tricky, Armstrong admits, because there's definitely a tendency for children to rebel against the ideas of their parents. "So I've really tried not to be overly aggressive with what we are feeding them or with any information I'm giving them," he says. "But just to show them. They are well aware of the effects of industrialized mass-produced sugars on the well-being of children across the nation. They know about

it. They've seen it in the media, too. It's not just Dad on another crazy rant."

Cardoz says, "I tell my kids what's in food. I tell them how it's processed. I tell them to read labels. My eleven-year-old reads labels on boxes himself now."

Armstrong and his wife are particular about snacks for the kids because they are mostly packaged foods, frequently loaded with ingredients like chemicals and refined sugars. He admits no child wants to eat "health food," and his strategy is to seek out healthier options like fruit leathers without chemicals and preservatives. "They don't have snacks available to them that are not healthy. They don't drink soda, but we use soda as a good reward, like if we are on vacation somewhere, they are allowed to have soda. Other than that they don't drink soda, and they are not that interested in soda." Of his kids Berley adds, "We never had soda in the house—ever. We never bought soda—it just didn't exist. Maybe they had soda when they were outside with their friends. They didn't have it at home."

Schmidt believes children crave sugary snacks, candy, and soda when they eat a lot of refined carbohydrates, and that moderation comes from not eating a lot of refined carbohydrates like white flour, white sugar, white rice, and low-protein white-flour pasta. He explains that when you eat refined carbohydrates, you burn through them, your sugar level drops, and you immediately crave more carbohydrates. He says that it takes four or five days of cutting back on eating refined carbohydrates for the body to assimilate the proteins and such differently, and then you won't crave those foods any longer. He keeps his children on a diet of low-glycemic foods and says of his kids, "They like their sweet stuff, but neither of them has a sweet tooth—they'd rather have fruit than a big chocolate cake or something like that."

When Hopkins makes biscuits, he uses lard, because as a Southerner, raised on biscuits, that's what belongs in biscuits. He says, "It's just a matter of, is it good lard? Were these happy pigs? My definition of good food is—well, ice cream is good for you. I don't really see a problem with real cream with farm eggs. We don't really serve dessert with our meals at home, but I have no problem with real ice cream or real cake or real cookies. I like my milk to be a single ingredient—on the back of the carton it reads 'milk.'"

Lunches—The Lure of Nuggets

"A kid will not eat broiled chicken every day," says Bromberg, "but she will eat nuggets five times a week!" Bromberg admits that lunches are complicated for him because at school the food is generally unhealthy, and while his children like eating some of the things served at school, some they don't. It's a balance, and he lets them choose. "Sometimes Jason likes triple-decker ham and cheese sandwiches with the crusts cut off. We make him those. My daughter, Leah, if she doesn't like her lunch, she just doesn't eat it. She'll come home from school, she'll say, 'I'm starving.'"

Bromberg's approach is to let them choose what they're going to do while offering guidance. His children read the school lunch menu that's published for the week, and together they focus on choosing the

B. T. NGUYEN is one of Tampa's most talented and best-known chefs. She sums up her culinary approach in three words: authentic, healthy, and fresh, and her hip French Vietnamese restaurant reflects her sensibilities, using local sources. She has a daughter, Trina, and a son, James. She says, "My daughter grew up in the restaurant business. We started as a very small restaurant, and I took Trina with me since she was a baby—she's always been around food. Her good eating habits started when she was young."

B.T. Nguyen and son James : NORMAN BATLEY

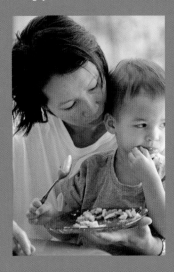

school lunches the kids like without too much focus on the nutritional aspect, because Bromberg recognizes that lunches in school are a social function. His children want to participate with their friends. Bromberg says, "They're in school and that's what's going on and they need to sit with everybody and go through the line. . . . There's a lot of peer pressure for so many things, and food is definitely one of them, especially because they all eat together as a group in school. There's only a small list of things on the school lunch menu that Leah will try."

Chef B. T. Nguyen says of her daughter, Trina, "She started packing her own lunch. But she wants to be cool. Like anybody she doesn't want to be controlled by her mother in what she eats. But she finds that the food at school is not good—it's canned food or frozen food. Her palate is extremely sophisticated. She eats raw oysters, raw tuna. She wants her beef medium rare. She really loves food. As much as she's trying to be cool, to fit in."

"For breakfasts, we kind of make it a variety of stuff," says Bromberg, "but we don't generally go for muffins and cakes and that kind of breakfast, because they kinda get really hyped up and then before lunch happens at school they're falling asleep or running around, crazy."

"You know people ask me about when my son used to have a peanut butter and jelly sandwich for school every day for lunch. That's what he used to like to eat. People say, is it true? Doesn't he get sick of it? Yeah, he liked that . . . it was a good peanut butter and a good jelly," says Citrin. He packs his kids school lunches. "I give them what they like," he says. "Today

SALLY KRAVICH is one of the leading natural health practitioners in the country. She holds a Master of Science in holistic nutrition and is currently completing her Ph.D. Her background spans a lifetime of studies, and she combines extensive global studies, firsthand experience of historical and cultural remedies, and a vast knowledge of food as medicine to support clients on the path of wellness and healthy living. Her unparalleled career provides guidance for uniting body, mind, and spirit. Widely regarded as an authority on health, vitality, and wellness, Sally's advice has been cited in *Harper's BAZAAR, W, Essence,* and many other magazines. She has been featured as a nutritional expert for pregnancy with Aleta St. James on NBC's *Dateline.* Her specialized programs integrate practical wisdom with modern methods for achieving vibrant, radiant health. Her approach is outlined in her book, *Vibrant Living: Creating Radiant Health and Longevity.* She also has a DVD series and is working on a cookbook for preparing fast, easy, healthful, delicious meals.

•• Use sauces. **"I find having a sauce in your food really helps,"** says Chef Linton Hopkins. He explains that at his house a little pan drippings left over from a roast chicken spooned on a side dish of rice goes over well. Sauces provide that delicious umami flavor to foods and can be a bit rich or a bit sweet.

•• Feed them when they are hungry. **Kids tend** to eat what's put in front of them more when they are hungry—not overly hungry but hungry.

•• Set a timetable for dining. **Children need** consistency in general, explains Chef Cathal Armstrong. He says that schedules are really helpful when raising children. Dinner is at six o'clock. It always has to be ready at six o'clock. He finds that when something's happened and dinner is pushed back, it's too late; his children are really too hungry, and they get cranky, making dinnertime difficult.

•• Control snacking. **If children are eating** dinner on a set schedule consistently, it's easier to control what time they have their snacks. If dinner becomes late, the first thing kids reach for are snacks that contain sugar, because sugar is the fastest source of energy, explains Armstrong. Then they have a sugar high, and then they crash again. It's all a big mess, he says.

•• Include important nutrients. **Health expert** Sally Kravich recommends calcium, B vitamins, and fish oil for children at this age, who are growing, beginning puberty, and consequently may have acne or become moody. She advises eating vegetables like bok choy, which are high in calcium, and supplementing with additional calcium and other helpful nutrients. She says to try to limit sugar, because it makes children more nervous and off balance.

what I did, I had some nice salami, I put some salami in his lunch, a bottle of water, I did a sliced cucumber for him, some carrots, some grapes—it's enough for him to choose."

This age is a gateway to being teenagers—children begin to read and acquire their own information and so formulate their own opinions. They begin to feel grown up and want to think for themselves and want to have some control over their lives. They still need real adult guidance, but having them participate in the choices and preparation of meals is even more important. It gives them a way to feel their choices and input are valued.

Hopkins says, "I'm trying to get them to pack their own lunch so that they start learning about choices. I'll watch what they pack and augment it with whatever I see it's lacking. My daughter loves tangerines and my son loves kumquats, so we make sure those are always available, and we'll invariably have around some kind of crackers and cheese. They can make sandwiches for themselves—peanut butter and jelly or turkey and cheese sandwiches. Yogurt is also popular. Radishes and little carrots and those kinds of things seem to be the most popular items."

potato chip–crusted chicken tenders

{ JOSIAH CITRIN }

SERVES 4

Chef Josiah Citrin recommends this recipe because it is interactive and the kids enjoy helping. They like the potato chips, so it's fun for them. Citrin suggests trying out different-flavored potato chips and trying them on pork cutlets and even crab cakes. The cutlets come out really crispy—crispier than when using bread crumbs. He recommends serving them with a salad of grated vegetables that the kids can also prepare or string beans. Leftover chicken makes great lunch sandwiches, or it can be frozen for a later date for heating quickly in the oven. I make extra to freeze for Cody on nights when we have a babysitter prepare dinner.

Hawaiian or other light-colored nonsalted potato chips
Egg white
3 chicken breasts
Lemon wedges or Mayonnaise Sauce (see page 181)

1. Grind up the potato chips by spreading them out on a cutting board and rolling over them with a rolling pin until they are finely ground. Consider placing them in a large, sealable plastic bag to keep the crumbs contained.

2. Place the egg white in a bowl (save the yolk for the Mayonnaise Sauce).

3. Cover each chicken breast with plastic wrap and pound it down with the smooth side of a meat mallet so it is a consistent thickness.

4. Preheat oven to 375°F.

5. Cut the cutlets into "tenders" and brush on the egg white.

6. Coat the chicken pieces well with the ground potato chips and bake in the oven on a foil-lined baking sheet until crispy, about 15 minutes, depending on the size and thickness of the chicken pieces.

7. Squeeze lemon on top or serve with Mayonnaise Sauce (recipe at right).

Mayonnaise Sauce:

1 egg yolk

1 teaspoon Dijon mustard

½ lemon, juiced

1 cup olive oil (do not use extra-virgin, it will become
bitter)

Water as necessary

1 ripe Roma tomato, diced

1. Combine egg yolk with mustard and lemon juice in a
bowl big enough to whisk all the ingredients together.

2. Slowly add the olive oil and whisk together until
the sauce gets thick, adding drops of water if it gets
too thick. Continue adding the oil in small quantities
and whisking until thick and blended.

3. Mix in diced tomato.

Notes: If you're concerned about the fat in the potato
chips, try cornflakes or coat only one side—cook
crusted-side down first.

You can cheat on the Mayonnaise Sauce by adding
Dijon mustard and lemon juice to a big dollop of jarred
mayonnaise.

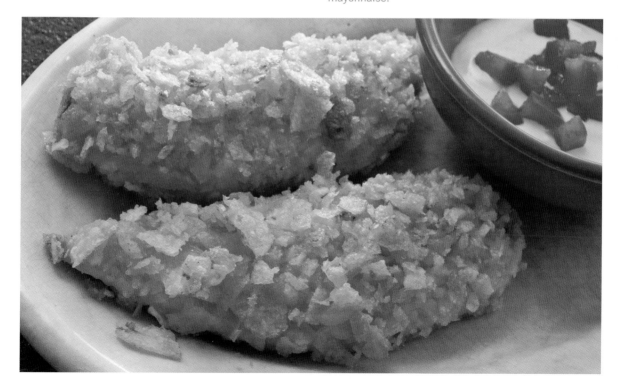

kalbi steak

{ JOSIAH CITRIN }

SERVES 4

This is the favorite meal at the Citrin household and a lunchbox hit. We make this for dinner and sometimes serve it in bowls and other times serve it with large lettuce leaves to make wraps and bundles at the table. I pack the leftover rice, steak, and vegetables for the next day's lunch for Cody. The marinade also works for pork and chicken.

Please note that this recipe calls for marinating the steak for several hours or overnight; plan accordingly.

Kalbi Marinade:

½ cup soy sauce

¼ cup water

2 tablespoons sesame oil

2 tablespoons rice vinegar

2½ tablespoons sugar

3 cloves garlic, pressed, crushed, or minced

2 teaspoons minced fresh ginger

2 tablespoons coarsely chopped onion

Steak:

16 ounces rib eye or NY strip or skirt steak, sliced
 ¼-inch thick

1 cup rice

1 tablespoon toasted sesame seeds, as garnish
 (optional)

2 green onions, as garnish (optional)

Vegetables such as shredded carrot or cabbage, thinly
 sliced daikon, or cucumber, for serving (optional)

1. Whisk all the marinade ingredients together until blended and the sugar has dissolved.

2. Pour a portion of the marinade into a smaller container and save for a dipping sauce. Combine the rest of the marinade and the steak slices in a nonreactive glass or plastic bowl to marinate for 2 hours at room temperature or 4 hours to overnight in the refrigerator.

3. Cook the rice according to the package instructions.

4. Heat a grill pan or a griddle over high heat and quickly grill each steak slice, keeping a close eye on them—the sugar in the marinade will burn quickly.

5. Once cooked, arrange the steak on a platter and sprinkle with the toasted sesame seeds and green onions. Arrange the rice in a serving bowl and the vegetables on another platter. Let each person construct a bowl of their own, with steak and vegetables atop the rice. Have the reserved marinade in a bowl at the table for dipping.

Note: To pack for lunch, arrange the sesame seed– and green onion–sprinkled steak alongside the rice and other vegetables, or pack them in separate containers, depending on what kind of containers you have available. If packed in a single container, items can portioned and separated with cupcake wrappers. The reserved marinade dipping sauce should be packed in a separate sealed container.

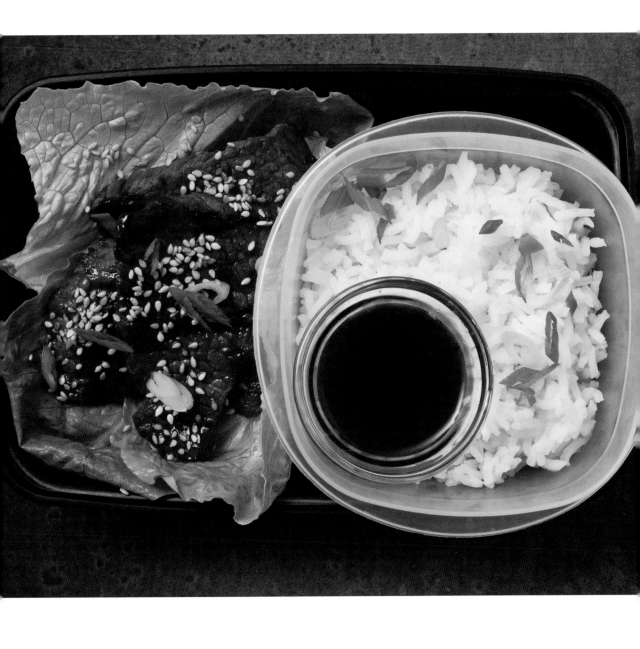

shaking beef

{ B. T. NGUYEN }

Chef B. T. Nguyen makes this dish, one of the most highly requested at her restaurant in Tampa, with good-quality beef and recommends using a Courvoisier cognac. Sometimes I buy the small single-serving bottles of cognac or other alcohol to use in recipes that call for small quantities of good-quality alcohol that I wouldn't necessarily have around for drinking. You can have the butcher cut the steak for you, or if you are doing it yourself, cut it when the meat is cold, with a sharp knife, and it will cut easier. While tasty made last minute, the dish is far better if you marinate the meat overnight—the meat gets a much deeper flavor. Double the marinade and save half to cook last minute in the wok for extra sauce. Serve with steamed jasmine rice. This recipe does require a bit of concentration and focus to get just right. I love watching my friend Piper make it—she tenderly watches and turns each piece of beef as it browns with chopsticks. The trick to this recipe is to cook the dish in small batches so that the beef gets seared on the outside and stays tender on the inside. Otherwise the pan or wok gets too crowded and beef will simmer in the sauce instead.

Note: This recipe calls for marinating for several hours or overnight; plan accordingly.

Marinade:

4 cloves garlic, finely chopped
1 tablespoon soy sauce
1 tablespoon fish sauce
1 tablespoon sugar
½ teaspoon freshly ground black pepper

Beef:

1 pound filet mignon or other similar tender cut, cut into bite-size cubes
1 tablespoon vegetable oil
1 tablespoon butter
Salt and pepper
¼ red onion, finely sliced
1½ tablespoons good-quality cognac
2 fresh ripe tomatoes, sliced
2 cups watercress (or arugula)

1. In a nonreactive bowl or container large enough to hold the beef, mix together all the marinade ingredients. Add the meat, mix to coat evenly, and let sit refrigerated for several hours or overnight.

2. Heat a large heavy-bottomed pan or wok until very hot, then add half the vegetable oil and swirl to coat the pan; next add half the butter. Turn and swirl the pan as the butter foams and turns a light

brown. Do not let the butter burn. Add half the beef cubes and toss with the oil by shaking the pan. Season with a pinch of salt and pepper. Let the meat sear for 2 minutes, then turn with tongs. Add half the sliced red onion and continue to cook the beef until seared on all sides but still a tender pink in the center. Repeat the steps with the other half of the ingredients.

3. Add the cognac for the last minute of cooking and shake the pan to release and coat the beef. Remove from heat.

4. To serve, arrange the tomato slices on plates and pile the watercress around or on top of the tomato slices. Place the beef in a mound on top of the tomatoes and watercress.

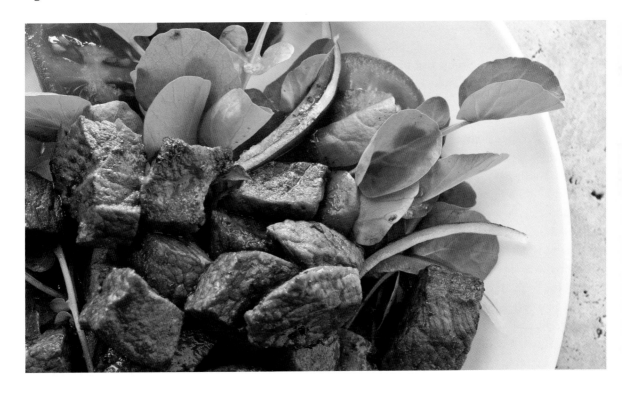

goan caldo verde

{ FLOYD CARDOZ }

SERVES 6

"We always have greens with our meals," says Chef Floyd Cardoz. "If I want them to eat kale, I do a soup with kale.... I use chorizo with potatoes and chicken stock, and then I puree the whole thing so it has the flavor of the chorizo and the flavor of the potato and so the kale is palatable."

When we make this soup we don't always puree it, and sometimes we add pasta because Cody, like most kids, loves pasta. He will eat only a little soup on its own, but he will fish out every last piece of pasta in the soup and, in the process, eat a good half bowl. Then, I pour the soup into a small cup so he can drink it. He thinks it's fun that way.

Chorizo has many varieties and all add a distinctive flavor to a dish. In Los Angeles the varieties readily available are either Spanish or Mexican, although chorizo also comes from South America, Portugal, Philippines, Dominican Republic, Puerto Rico, and Goan, India. Spanish chorizo is usually a cured smoked sausage, red from the dried smoked red peppers mixed in with the pork. Its flavor is distinctive, and it's usually eaten sliced without further cooking. Mexican chorizo is usually raw, with the texture of ground beef. It is also red from its high chile and spice content.

For added flavor, boil the kale in chicken or vegetable stock instead of water. You can save the stock afterwards to use again.

2 tablespoons canola oil

3 cloves

Bay leaf

1 tablespoon cumin seeds

1 teaspoon whole black peppercorns

½ cinnamon stick

½ cup sliced onions

5 cloves garlic, sliced

2 cups chorizo or similar sausage, sliced

2 cups canned diced tomatoes

1 cup diced celery root

2 cups peeled, diced potatoes

2 quarts chicken stock

Salt

Pepper

½ pound kale, washed, stemmed, and cut into thick strips (or substitute spinach)

Pasta (optional)

1. In a heavy-bottomed 6-quart Dutch oven or soup pot, heat the canola oil over medium heat. Add the cloves, bay leaf, cumin, black pepper, and cinnamon stick and cook until fragrant, about 3 minutes.

2. Next, add the sliced onions and garlic and cook over medium-low heat for 5 minutes, until softened and transparent.

3. Add the sausage and when browned, add the tomatoes and celery root and cook for 4 minutes more.

4. Add potatoes and the stock, bring to a boil, reduce to a simmer, and cook for 30 minutes, until tender. Season to taste with salt and pepper.

5. Bring a medium pot of water to a boil, then add 1 tablespoon salt. When the water returns to a boil, add the kale a handful at a time and cook for 2 to 3 minutes until the kale is tender but still bright green. Remove with a spoon and cool. Continue to cook each batch this way until all the kale is cooked.

6. Remove the bay leaf from the soup. You can either stir in the kale and serve with pasta (optional) or puree and serve.

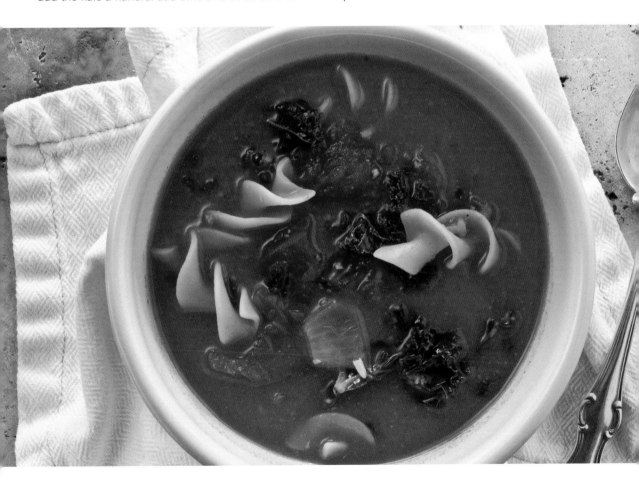

baked halibut with potatoes and tomatoes

{ JOSIAH CITRIN }

SERVES 4

This is a great way to introduce kids to fish. Halibut has a delicate flavor and the cornflakes sprinkled on top give it a crunch that kids will love to pick off and eat. Sometimes children need a way into a dish, and the familiar crunch of the cornflake topping gives them just that. A child serving is half a fillet. Chef Josiah Citrin recommends serving with jasmine rice.

12 or so fingerling potatoes

Butter for coating the baking dish

4 6-ounce halibut fillets (or any mild white fish),
   skinned and deboned

Salt and pepper

1 lemon, juiced

1 tablespoon olive oil

Approximately 1 cup water

12 cherry tomatoes

5 fresh basil leaves, chopped

1 teaspoon Dijon mustard

¼ cup cornflakes crushed into large crumbs

1. Boil the potatoes until just tender, about 15 minutes depending on their freshness, and slice ½-inch thick.

2. Preheat oven to 350°F.

3. Butter a baking dish large enough to hold all the halibut fillets in one layer, and lay the fillets in the dish, leaving a bit of room between the fillets and around the edge of the dish. Sprinkle the fish with salt and pepper and squeeze the lemon juice over the fillets.

4. Drizzle the olive oil and add enough water to the pan to come halfway up the thickness of the fish. Scatter the potato slices and the whole cherry tomatoes along the edge of the baking dish and sprinkle the basil leaves all over on top.

5. Cover with parchment paper or aluminum foil and put the baking dish in the oven to bake slowly for 15 to 20 minutes, until the fish is just cooked through and still moist.

6. Remove the dish from the oven and brush the top of the fish with mustard and sprinkle lightly with the cornflakes (do not cover the whole fillets). Place the dish quickly in the broiler for just 20 seconds for the crumbs to get crunchy but not burnt.

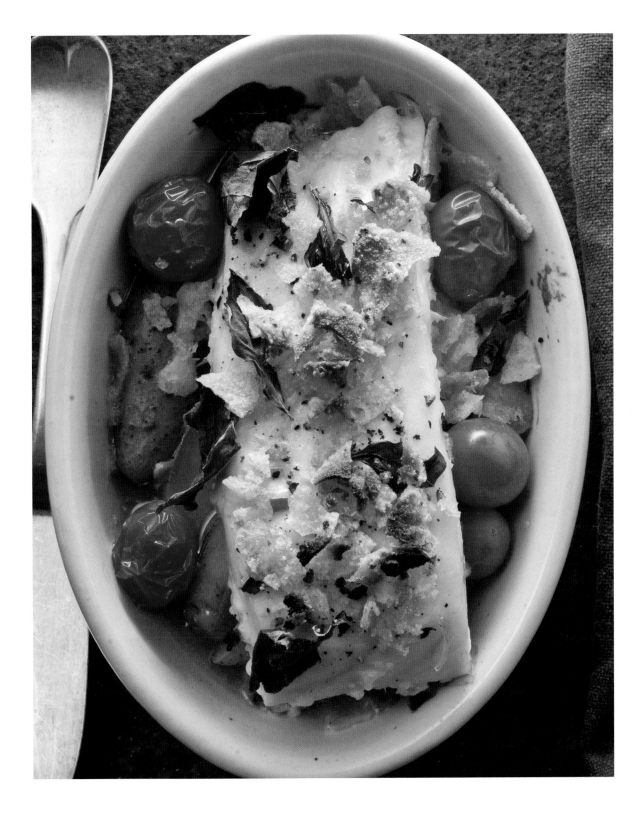

goan shrimp curry

{ FLOYD CARDOZ }

SERVES 6

I always welcome making an interesting one-pot dish like this shrimp curry. Make sure to shake the can of coconut milk before opening and pouring it in the dish.

2 pounds peeled shrimp

Salt

½ teaspoon black pepper

1 teaspoon cumin

1 cup shredded coconut

6 cloves garlic

4 cups shrimp stock or water, divided

1 teaspoon turmeric

2 tablespoons tamarind paste

2 tablespoons canola oil

¾ cup onion, sliced

2 fresh chile peppers, split (Anaheim work well)

1 can coconut milk, well shaken before pouring

Sea salt

1. Season the shrimp with salt and let stand for between 15 and 30 minutes in the refrigerator.

2. Grind the pepper and cumin in a spice grinder until finely ground.

3. Combine the coconut and garlic in a blender cup with 1 cup shrimp stock or water. Blend until smooth and combine with the mixture of spices, the turmeric, and the tamarind paste.

4. Place a medium-size pot over medium heat. Add the canola oil; when hot add the sliced onions and sauté for 3 to 4 minutes. Next add the spice paste and cook for 2 to 3 minutes. Add the remaining 3 cups of stock or water, chiles, coconut milk, and sea salt and cook over medium-low heat, stirring and not letting the liquid boil, for 10 to 15 minutes.

5. Cook the shrimp in the sauce until just done and still tender, approximately 10 minutes, stirring every now and again.

Tip: If you have a bit of time, make your own shrimp stock from the shells. Simply peel the shrimp and add the shells to a pot with water (for 2 pounds shrimp use 2 quarts water). Add an onion; some celery and carrot; and some herbs, like parsley, thyme, and a bay leaf. Make sure to skim the surface as the stock cooks. It will take about an hour to cook, but it smells delicious and will add much more flavor to the dish.

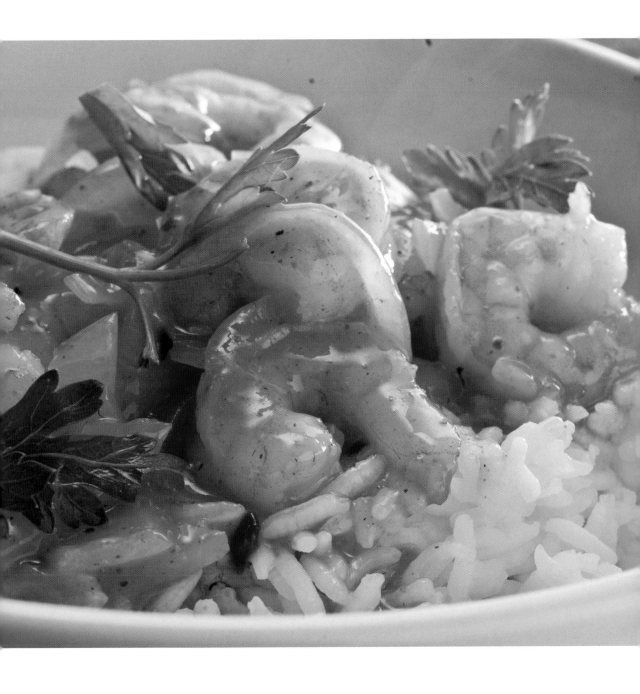

lemongrass snapper

{ B. T. NGUYEN }

"The fresher the ingredients, the better the food," says Chef B. T. Nguyen. If you prep the fish so it's ready to go in the morning or the night before, this is a superfast dinner served simply with rice or with Lemongrass Risotto (page 198).

Note: **This recipe calls for marinating for several hours or overnight; plan accordingly.**

1 3-pound whole red snapper or yellowtail, or 2 smaller fish, preferably butted, cleaned, and deboned

1–2 stalks fresh lemongrass, tough outer leaves removed and discarded, interior chopped fine or pureed

1 dried bay leaf, crumbled, or 1 fresh bay leaf, chopped

1 teaspoon grated fresh galangal or ½ teaspoon grated fresh ginger

1 garlic glove, sliced

1½ teaspoons mild curry powder

1½ teaspoons vegetable oil

1½ teaspoons soy sauce

1 teaspoon sugar

⅛ teaspoon black pepper or more to taste

1. Clean the fish, including the cavity, in fresh water and pat dry. Make three medium cuts on the outside of both sides of the fish and set aside.

2. In a small food processor or mortar and pestle, mix the lemongrass, bay leaf, galangal or ginger, garlic, curry powder, vegetable oil, soy sauce, sugar, and black pepper and pulse or pound into a paste. The lemongrass stalks are fibrous, so make sure to pound well until softened or puree well.

3. Using your hands, rub the spice mixture into the cavity of the fish and into the cuts on the outside of the fish.

4. Wrap the fish tightly in plastic wrap and marinate in the refrigerator for at least 3 hours.

5. When ready to cook, heat oven to 450°F. Unwrap the fish and bake on a tray or in a ceramic dish in the oven for 25 minutes or until done.

Note: Lemongrass stalks have a lovely elusive flavor but are fibrous and can be hard to prepare correctly, especially for young kids. It works best to cut the yellow section of the stalk into thin slices and grind them in a mini grinder/chopper or food processor that handles small quantities, adding a bit of water or oil if necessary. For very small amounts, pound with a mortar and pestle. If preparing in a soup, the lemongrass will soften as the soup simmers.

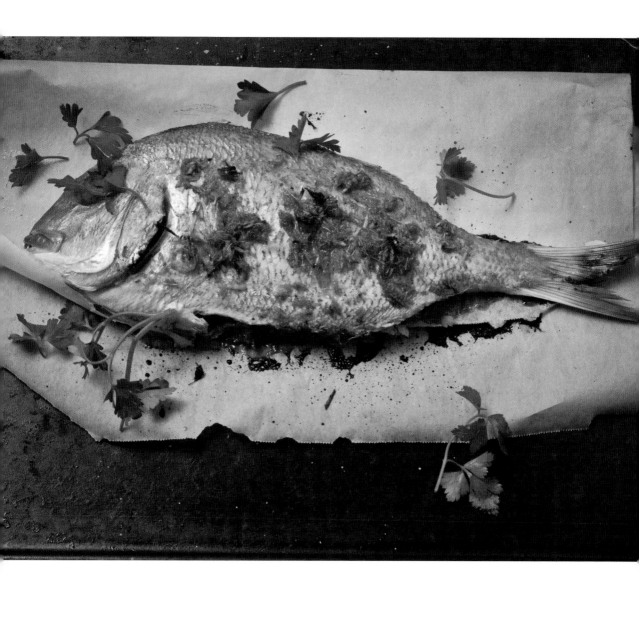

gratins of squash

{ LINTON HOPKINS }

Most gratins are baked with cream or milk and lots of cheese. In the summertime, when squash is so abundant, Chef Linton Hopkins makes lighter gratins with summer squash simply dressed with olive oil, onion, and Parmesan cheese. The squash stays brightly colored and is tender without being overcooked and mushy. Sometimes we add garlic with the onion or add a layer of tomatoes to the gratin, or sometimes we add some fresh basil or marjoram.

1 pound yellow or green summer squash, thinly sliced
1 teaspoon kosher salt
1½ teaspoons olive oil, divided
½ Vidalia or other sweet mild onion, chopped
Salt and pepper
½ cup grated Parmesan cheese, divided

1. Lay the sliced squash in a colander; massage the salt onto the squash, and let sit for 20 minutes, until beads of sweat form. Rinse the squash under water and pat dry.

2. Preheat oven to 350°F.

3. Heat a sauté pan over medium heat, and, when hot, add 1 teaspoon olive oil. Add the Vidalia onions and sauté until soft and translucent, about 4 minutes. While onion cooks, in a bowl combine and mix the squash with remaining ½ teaspoon olive oil plus salt and pepper.

4. To assemble the gratin, cover the bottom of the baking dish with about ⅓ of the sautéed onions. Arrange about ⅓ of the squash slices on top, and sprinkle about ⅓ of the cheese over the squash. Repeat layers two more times and top with a thicker blanket of cheese.

5. Bake uncovered for 25 minutes, until the squash has softened, the cheese has melted, and the top has turned a golden brown.

Note: Vidalia onions are sweet yellow onions grown in Georgia. They are juicy and flavorful and sweet enough to be eaten raw. Buy what you need and use them quickly, as they don't store well.

summer tomato fondue

{ LINTON HOPKINS }

SERVES 4 AS A LIGHT SIDE DISH

"We really try to celebrate the ingredients," says Chef Linton Hopkins. He makes a tomato fondue all the time in the summer, when tomatoes are piled high at the markets and incredibly flavorful. Tomato fondue can be served on toast, over fish or lentils, or plain on a plate, next to some meat or fish. It can be cooked long and slow to make it richer and thicker; butter and roasted garlic or herbs can be added to round out the flavor.

2 tablespoons olive oil

¼ onion, chopped

3 pints cherry tomatoes, cut in half or quarters, or use another fresh ripe tomato cut in pieces

Salt and pepper

Sugar to taste

Fresh basil or other fresh herbs like parsley or tarragon, chopped (optional)

1 tablespoon butter (optional)

1. Heat a medium sauté pan on medium-low heat; add the olive oil to warm. Add the chopped onions, stir, and cover to soften the onions but not brown them, about 5 minutes.

2. Raise the heat, add the tomatoes, and cook for several minutes over moderately high heat until the tomatoes have cooked down and the juice has thickened a bit, about 5 minutes.

3. Season the tomatoes with salt and pepper, add a sprinkle of sugar if needed, and mix in herbs and butter, if you like.

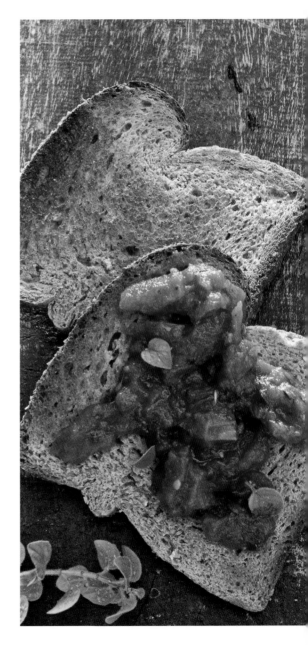

cast-iron charred cherry tomatoes and squash blossoms

{ CHRIS COSENTINO }

SERVES 4

Cody had never eaten squash blossoms, and I'd never cooked them before. I admit I was a bit scared to eat them; they are unusual looking. Cody, too, was hesitant. To encourage him to try these, I made a fun game out of it—we would count to three and then eat. His eyes got wide with surprise—and so did mine—at how good they tasted, from the blossom to the crunchy stem. We ate them all that way, down to the last one, which we split. This will become our springtime favorite. Have all your ingredients together, as this cooks very fast. The goal is to char the tomatoes without having them break apart. You will need a very hot burner to cook this on the stovetop.

1½ pints mixed cherry tomatoes
12 squash blossoms with stems attached
1½ teaspoon extra-virgin olive oil
Maldon sea salt or other sea salt
2 tablespoons basil (piccolo fino preferred)
Black pepper

1. Heat a large cast-iron pan over the center of a fire or on the highest setting of the hottest burner on your stove.

2. While the pan is heating, wash the tomatoes and squash blossoms, being sure to leave the stems on the blossoms (they're delicious), and remove the stamen from the center of the squash blossoms.

3. Once the pan is screaming hot, add the olive oil, then throw in all the cherry tomatoes and blossoms, season with Maldon salt, and then add the basil. Once the basil is added, remove from flame, season to taste with black pepper, and serve immediately.

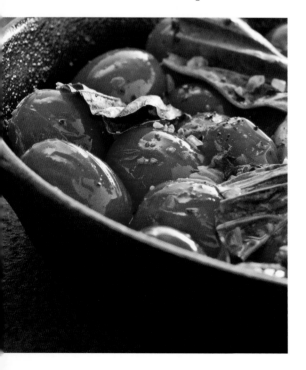

corn cakes

{ LINTON HOPKINS }

SERVES 4

Corn cakes, also known as johnnycakes, are a simply made down-home savory cross between corn bread and pancakes, delicious served with chili or soup or fancied up with lemon zest and honey and served warm with crème fraîche and jam or fresh berries. Chef Linton Hopkins makes them by adding buttermilk to cornmeal with a touch of salt. There's no one way to make corn cakes. Instead it's better to flavor them as needed for what you're serving. Add some chives and fresh corn for serving with sour cream as a side dish for a dinner entree, or make them sweeter if serving for breakfast.

Tips: Wipe out the pan between batches when cooking to remove any burned butter, which has an unpleasant taste. See page 109 for a quick substitute for buttermilk.

½ cup cornmeal

½ cup flour

1 teaspoon salt

¾ teaspoon baking powder

¼ teaspoon baking soda

½ cup buttermilk (plus more for thinning)

2 tablespoons honey or sorghum molasses

1 egg

1 tablespoon butter

1. Whisk together cornmeal, flour, salt, baking powder, and baking soda in a bowl. In a saucepan, heat the buttermilk and honey or molasses together over low heat until the honey is melted. Pour the mixture slowly over the cornmeal mixture, whisking to prevent lumps. Add a bit more buttermilk to thin the batter if necessary; then add the egg.

2. Butter a large skillet or griddle and heat to medium heat. Grease a spoon with a bit of oil and scoop tablespoons of batter into the pan; spread and flatten a bit with the back of the spoon.

3. Let the cakes gently cook until they are a deep golden brown on the bottom and a bit firm on the edges, about 2 or so minutes depending on how thick and big they are, and then turn them over like regular pancakes.

4. Spread a bit more butter on the griddle and on each cake before turning them over and cooking for another 6 minutes (or longer), until they are a deep golden brown and cooked through. Corn cakes are best served warm, but they can be added to lunchboxes or refrigerated for another snack or meal.

lemongrass risotto

{ B. T. NGUYEN }

SERVES 4

This risotto is uniquely made without cheese. The shiitake mushrooms add a wonderful flavor, and you don't miss the creaminess the cheese would add otherwise.

Note: Lemongrass stalks have a lovely elusive flavor but are fibrous and can be hard to prepare correctly. It works best to cut the yellow section of stalk into thin slices and ground them either in a food processor or pound them until soft with a mortar and pestle. If preparing in a soup or risotto, as for this recipe, the lemongrass will soften as it cooks.

6 cups chicken, fish, or vegetable stock
Salt and pepper
3 tablespoons canola oil, olive oil, or butter
1 large onion, diced
3 stalks fresh lemongrass, finely chopped
1 carrot, diced
1 cup leeks, diced
1⅔ cups Arborio or jasmine rice
¾ cup dry white wine
1 cup shiitake mushrooms, stems removed and tops sliced
1 tablespoon fish sauce

1. In a medium saucepan, heat the stock, season with salt and pepper if needed, and keep warm over a very low flame.

2. Heat oil or butter in a large nonreactive saucepan, add onion, lemongrass, carrots, and leeks; cook over high heat for 3 minutes.

3. Add rice and sauté for 3 more minutes.

4. Once the rice starts to become translucent, add the white wine and shiitake mushrooms and stir. Cook until the wine is all absorbed; then add the stock ladle by ladle, making sure the liquid is absorbed before adding the next ladle, and stirring constantly. Continue until the rice is al dente, about 20 to 25 minutes, stirring frequently until all the liquid is absorbed.

5. Add fish sauce, mix well. Taste for seasoning, add salt and pepper as necessary, and serve.

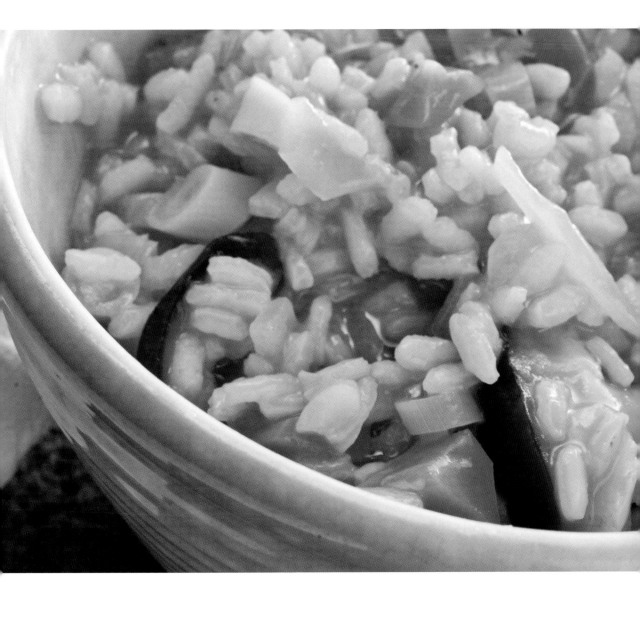

risotto with pumpkin, ginger, and sage

{ PETER BERLEY }

SERVES 4 WITH LEFTOVERS

I'm always looking for ways to cook pumpkin in the fall when Halloween is all around—it always feels festive and comforting. If pumpkin season has passed, try using sweet potatoes or winter squash.

2 tablespoons extra-virgin olive oil

1 cup finely chopped leek (white part only)

3 cups peeled pumpkin or winter squash, cut in
   ½-inch cubes (about 1 pound)

1 tablespoon peeled and minced fresh ginger

5 cups water or vegetable stock

Sea salt

Freshly ground black pepper

1 tablespoon finely chopped fresh sage

1½ cups Arborio rice

½ cup dry white wine

2 tablespoons unsalted butter

½ cup finely grated Parmesan cheese

3 teaspoons finely chopped parsley

½ cup toasted pumpkin seeds (recipe at right)

1. In large sauté pan, heat the olive oil over medium heat and, when warm, add the leeks, pumpkin or squash, and ginger and sauté for 5 minutes.

2. Meanwhile, heat the water or stock in a pot and season with salt and pepper if needed; keep warm over a low flame.

3. In the sauté pan, stir in the sage and rice. Once the rice starts to become translucent, add the white wine and stir. Cook until the wine is all absorbed; then add the stock ladle by ladle, being sure the liquid is absorbed before adding the next ladle, and stirring frequently. Continue until the rice is al dente, about 20 to 25 minutes.

4. Add the butter and cook, stirring with a wooden spoon, for 1 to 2 minutes, then stir in the cheese.

5. Turn off the heat and let the risotto rest, uncovered, for 3 minutes before serving.

6. Add sea salt and freshly ground pepper to taste. Serve sprinkled with parsley and Toasted Pumpkin Seeds (recipe follows).

Toasted Pumpkin Seeds:

½ cup pumpkin seeds (shelled)

½ teaspoon extra-virgin olive oil

Pinch fine sea salt

1. Preheat oven to 375°F.

2. In a bowl, toss the seeds, oil, and salt together. Spread the seeds on a cookie sheet and toast in the oven for 15 minutes. Cool until crisp.

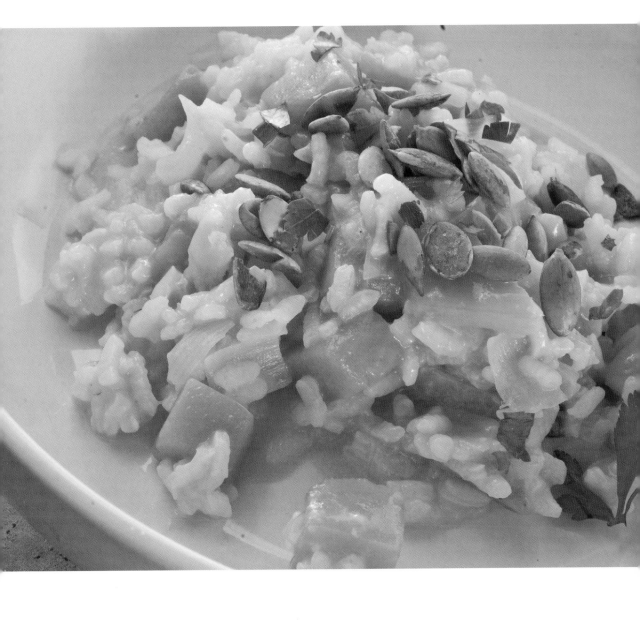

homemade ranch dressing

{ LINTON HOPKINS }

MAKES ABOUT 1 CUP

This dressing thickens up after a bit in the fridge—perfect for dipping veggies in. For an even thicker dressing, add extra sour cream and use a thick Greek-style yogurt.

1 small clove garlic, minced

¼ teaspoon salt

¼ cup sour cream or crème fraîche or thick plain
    yogurt

¼ cup mayonnaise

2 tablespoons buttermilk (plus more for thinning)

½ teaspoon white wine vinegar or lemon juice

1 tablespoon chopped fresh parsley

½ tablespoon chopped fresh dill

½ teaspoon chopped chives

Salt and pepper to taste

1. Mash the minced garlic and salt with a mortar and pestle to make a paste.

2. In a bowl, combine the garlic paste with the sour cream, crème fraîche, or yogurt; mayonnaise; and buttermilk. Add more buttermilk to thin for a pourable dressing or less for a dip.

3. Add the vinegar and herbs and season with salt and pepper. The dressing will store refrigerated for several days. The flavors will meld and get better; stir again before serving.

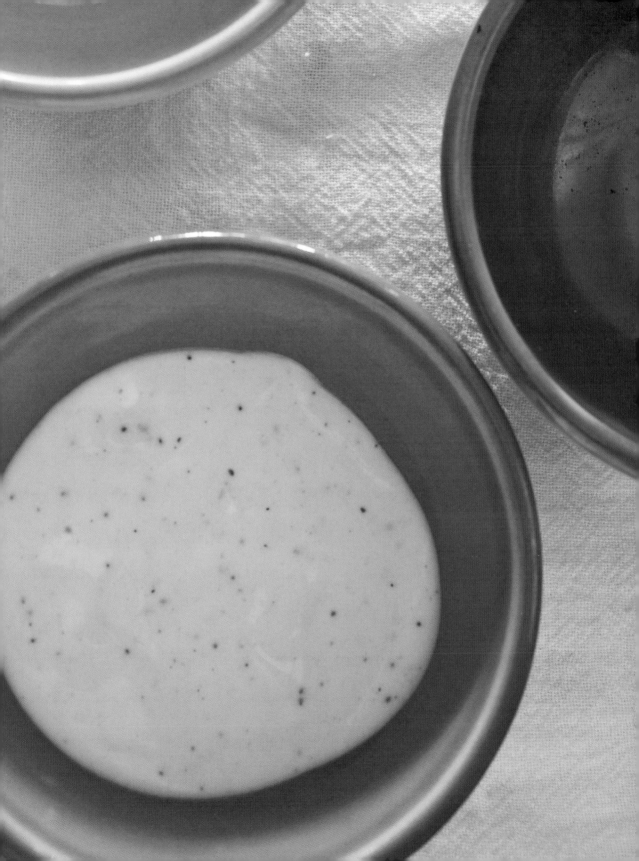

lemon bars

{ JOAN MCNAMARA }

MAKES 9 BARS

These lemon bars are signature treats at Chef Joan McNamara's Los Angeles food emporium, Joan's on Third. It's hard to resist these pretty lemony treats, dusted with sugar and just the right balance of tart and sweet. She says she always had lemon bars in the freezer ready for her kids when they had friends over. It made hers the favorite house to visit.

½ cup (1 stick) butter, melted
1¼ cups flour, divided
Pinch salt
½ cup sugar
½ teaspoon baking powder
2 eggs, slightly beaten
¾ cup honey
2 teaspoons lemon zest
5 tablespoons fresh lemon juice
Powdered sugar for dusting the bars

1. Heat oven to 350°F.

2. To make the crust, combine the melted butter with 1 cup flour, salt, and the sugar in a medium bowl and mix until a dough forms. Press dough into an 8-inch square pan, leaving a thicker edge to make a sturdy crust for the filling. Bake until lightly browned, about 18 minutes. Remove from the oven and cool. Leave the oven on.

3. For the custard filling, mix together the remaining ¼ cup flour and baking powder in a medium bowl. In another bowl, beat together the eggs, honey, lemon zest, and lemon juice. Whisk the egg mixture into the flour mixture until combined. Pour into the baked crust and put back in the oven to bake for 20 to 25 minutes, until the filling is set. Remove and cool.

4. When cooled completely, dust lightly with powdered sugar and cut into bars.

Note: Lemon bars will keep in the refrigerator for 1 week, or can be frozen on a baking tray and then stored between layers of parchment or waxed paper in an airtight container. Simply defrost and serve.

Tip: You can easily make just the right amount of your own powdered sugar by putting regular granulated sugar in a blender or food processor.

metric conversion tables

Metric U.S. Approximate Equivalents

Liquid Ingredients

METRIC	U.S. MEASURES	METRIC	U.S. MEASURES
1.23 ML	1/4 TSP.	29.57 ML	2 TBSP.
2.36 ML	1/2 TSP.	44.36 ML	3 TBSP.
3.70 ML	3/4 TSP.	59.15 ML	1/4 CUP
4.93 ML	1 TSP.	118.30 ML	1/2 CUP
6.16 ML	1 1/4 TSP.	236.59 ML	1 CUP
7.39 ML	1 1/2 TSP.	473.18 ML	2 CUPS OR 1 PT.
8.63 ML	1 3/4 TSP.	709.77 ML	3 CUPS
9.86 ML	2 TSP.	946.36 ML	4 CUPS OR 1 QT.
14.79 ML	1 TBSP.	3.79 L	4 QTS. OR 1 GAL.

Dry Ingredients

METRIC	U.S. MEASURES	METRIC		U.S. MEASURES
2 (1.8) G	1/16 OZ.	80 G		2 4/5 OZ.
3 1/2 (3.5) G	1/8 OZ.	85 (84.9) G		3 OZ.
7 (7.1) G	1/4 OZ.	100 G		3 1/2 OZ.
15 (14.2) G	1/2 OZ.	115 (113.2) G		4 OZ.
21 (21.3) G	3/4 OZ.	125 G		4 1/2 OZ.
25 G	7/8 OZ.	150 G		5 1/4 OZ.
30 (28.3) G	1 OZ.	250 G		8 7/8 OZ.
50 G	1 3/4 OZ.	454 G	1 LB.	16 OZ.
60 (56.6) G	2 OZ.	500 G	1 LIVRE	17 3/5 OZ.

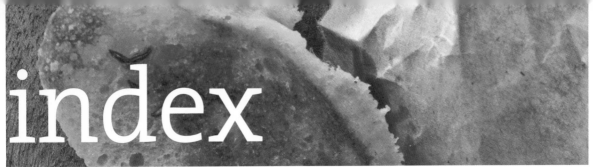

index

about the author

Trained in architecture and design, Fanae Aaron has worked as an art director for films and commercials with some of the most talented and creative people in the film industry. A lifelong interest in food and cooking was spurred on by the birth of her son Cody. Aaron grew up in New York City and now lives in Los Angeles with her husband Flint and Cody.